T0214805

Maternal Healthcare and Doulas in China

Zoe Z. Dai

Maternal Healthcare and Doulas in China

Health Communication Approach to Understanding Doulas in China

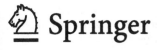 Springer

Zoe Z. Dai
School of Communication
Radford University
Radford, VA, USA

ISBN 978-3-030-46962-7   ISBN 978-3-030-46963-4   (eBook)
https://doi.org/10.1007/978-3-030-46963-4

This Springer imprint is published by the registered company Springer Nature Switzerland AG
The registered company address is: Gewerbestrasse 11, 6330 Cham, Switzerland

Preface

Many health scholars and practitioners believe that women who have had an embodied knowledge of the process have always supported other women in labor and childbirth. Since the 1990s, in the Chinese context, there has been an emergence of the "doula" phenomenon (Cheung, 2009). Some women have started to call themselves "doulas" and have been charging money for the support services that they provide during child labor. This revival of the role of the "doula" in the child birthing process is also visible in Western nations (Papagni & Buckner, 2006). According to Doulas of North America International (hereafter DONA), doulas are nonmedical maternal healthcare workers who provide physical, emotional, and informational support during pregnancy, childbirth, and/or the postpartum period (What is a doula, 2018). A doula's role is to help one birthing mother[1] to have a safe and comfortable childbirth experience by centering the birthing mother's body and feelings and by making sure that the birthing mother is able to holistically experience the childbirth process (Gruber et al., 2013; Hunter & Hurst, 2016).

As a research of health communication, I would like to focus this project broadly around an examination of the emergence of the doula phenomenon and the role that the doula workers play in the context of struggles for women's autonomy in the contexts of pregnancy and childbirth in China. I look at post-1980s contexts of midwifery—referred to as "doula care"—and how it is manifested in China. Doula and doula workers are a group of maternal healthcare workers. The doula care phenomenon—as it emerges as a viable profession for women in China—reveals nuances and contradictions and lends itself to an examination through a health communication lens and a relational communication perspective.

Radford, VA, USA   Zoe Z. Dai

---

[1] The terms expectant mother, pregnant woman, and birthing mother are used synonymously throughout the text. I am aware that since 2017 the British Medical Association has suggested health practitioners should use the phrase "pregnant people" instead of "expectant mothers" in order to show sensitivity toward intersex men and trans men who get pregnant. However, all the participants are female (sex)/women (gender) in this project. Hence, I use both the terms "expectant mother" and "pregnant woman" in this project instead of "pregnant people."

References

Cheung, N. F. (2009). Chinese midwifery: The history and modernity. *Midwifery, 25*(3), 228–241.

Gruber, K. J., Cupito, S. H., & Dobson, C. F. (2013). Impact of doulas on healthy birth outcomes. *The Journal of Perinatal Education, 22*(1), 49–58. https://doi.org/10.1891/1058-1243.22.1.49

Hunter, C. A., & Hurst, A. (2016). *Understanding doulas and childbirth: Women, love, and advocacy.* New York: Palgrave Macmillan. https://doi.org/10.1057/978-1-137-48536-48562.

Papagni, K., & Buckner, E. (2006). Doula support and attitudes of intrapartum nurses: A qualitative study from the patient's perspective. *The Journal of Perinatal Education, 15*(1), 11–18. https://doi.org/10.1624/105812406X92949

Acknowledgments

First and foremost, thanks to all my interviewees and many doulas, midwives, lactation consultants, and childbirth educators who supported me in this project. Thanks for sharing your insights, stories, happiness, and sorrows with me, in particular Dr. Jeannette T. Crenshaw, Shujuan, Suwan, Qian, and Qingrou. You are my DOULAS! Moreover, I would like to thank all the obstetrics staff at WeCare Women's Maternity Hospital.[1] The internship opportunity has helped me to understand the meaning of maternal healthcare in general. I appreciate and respect all the obstetrics staff who have worked (and are still working) very hard in their positions in order to provide respectful maternal healthcare for pregnant women and birthing mothers.

Furthermore, this book is written based on my doctoral dissertation project. Therefore, a heartful THANK YOU to my doctoral mentor and adviser Dr. Gajjala who worked with me in the past few years, with writing, talking, walking, coffee, and food. Thank you for your support! Thank you for being the extraordinary Spinning Professor! The book cannot be written without the support from my dissertation committee members, Drs. Gonzalez, Hanasono, and Hewitt. Importantly, many thanks also go to my academic sisters and friends, Drs. Jiang, Detteh, Han, and Feng. All of you are productive and amazing scholars. There is no doubt that your dissertations and publications have significant impacts on me. Meanwhile, I am grateful to have so many wonderful and supportive colleagues at my current working institution.

This book is dedicated to my open-minded and knowledgeable parents, who are my role models. Thanks for your unconditional support, trust, and love. I am privileged to be your daughter. Hopefully, I have not disappointed my parents since I did not graduate from a medical school and work as *a real doctor/physician*. Unfortunately, both of my grandfathers passed away before this book was officially published. Grandpa D and Grand H, we miss you!

---

[1] WeCare Women's Maternity Hospital is the research site of this project. I use pseudonyms for the maternity hospital of my research site in order to maintain confidentiality.

Contents

Chapter 1
Introduction

Doulas and Doula Care

A woman's ability to influence what she can do in the delivery room in most hospitals' childbirth settings is limited. Normally, obstetricians and midwives are in charge of the childbirth process and exert medical authority over the pregnant woman ready to give birth. However, as some health scholars have noted, ensuring a woman's ability to obtain respectful maternity healthcare and her ability to advocate for herself during labor are important (Kennedy, 2000, 2014). In fact, many health scholars and practitioners believe that women who have had an embodied knowledge of the process have always supported other women in labor and childbirth.

Doula is a Greek-derived term for a woman[1] who is experienced in providing continuous non-medical, physical, emotional, and informational support during pregnancy, childbirth, and/or the postpartum period (Stein et al., 2004; Dundek, 2006; Campbell et al., 2006; Gentry et al., 2010). The role of a doula is described as focusing on the pregnant woman's comfort and wishes during labor (Papagni & Buckner, 2006). A doula's role is fivefold: (1) to provide continuous emotional support (e.g., talking to the mother, providing encouragement with eye contact); (2) to keep the mother informed during the labor process; (3) to assist the mother to adopt particular birth-friendly physical positions during labor (e.g., liberal body positions); (4) to continuously communicate with the pregnant woman through verbal and non-verbal communication and to not let the mother feel alone; and (5) to facilitate immediate skin-to-skin touch between mother and baby following the birth and

---

[1] Theoretically, the term "sex" refers to biological profiles, and the term "gender" describes the characteristics that a society or culture delineates as masculine or feminine. The term "gender" also refers to social roles based on the sex of the person. I am aware that an individual's assigned sex and gender may not align, and the person may be transgender. Regarding the definition of "doulas" in current studies, they often refer to female (sex)/women (gender).

to promote breastfeeding (Tips for finding doula, 2018; Lamaze International Childbirth, 2017; Neifert & Seacat, 1986; Klaus et al., 2002; Langer et al., 1998; Stange et al., 2011).

The popularity of doula care has increased since the 1980s in the United States when researchers and health practitioners began to document the benefits of this kind of support during childbirth (Morton & Clift, 2014). Thousands of women have embraced this profession both in the United States and beyond (Kozhimannil et al., 2013; Steel et al., 2015). DONA International, founded in 1992, is the first and largest doula-recognized certifying organization in the United States and has more than 12,000 registered members (About DONA international, 2018). In addition, there are many other national and international organizations that train and certify doulas (e.g., International Childbirth Education Association, Childbirth Professions International; Childbirth and Postpartum Professional Association).

Doulas are unique since they are employed by pregnant women, but they have no medical decision-making responsibilities for birthing mothers (Davis-Floyd, 2004; Hodnett et al., 2007). They are expected to devote themselves and work throughout the entire childbirth process (Gilliland, 2002; Kennedy, 2014; Stein et al., 2004). The provision of doulas' caring work is varied. Some doulas provide assistance during labor and childbirth, and postpartum doulas provide care at the time after birth. Some doulas offer support for women who have abortions, miscarriages, and other reproductive experiences (Chor et al., 2012). Some doulas are in private practice and are paid by individuals for their services. Other doulas work on a volunteer basis, sometimes in formalized hospital-based programs designed to provide doula care to any women who may need labor support (Morton & Clift, 2014; Kozhimannil et al., 2016; Field observations, May 17, 2017).

Generally, there are three types of support that doulas provide for birthing mothers: emotional, physical, and informational support (Doula Training and Doula Certification [DONA], 2018; Klaus et al., 2002; Kozhimannil et al., 2013). Therefore, a doula's presence is simultaneously a critique of and a solution to the current maternity health system's lack of focus on women's emotional well-being during childbirth (Dahlen et al., 2011; He, 2011; Kayne et al., 2001). Doulas come from a wide variety of personal backgrounds, birthing experiences, and subscribe to varied maternity healthcare philosophies. It is important to point out that doulas' provision for birthing mothers is about non-judgmental support, and the purpose of doula care support aims to empower women in labor physically and psychologically (Amram et al., 2014; Dahlen et al., 2011; Hunter & Hurst, 2016).

Researchers have found that doula care encourages positive birth outcomes, including decreased need for medical technological interventions and pain medications (Hodnett et al., 2007) as well as lower rates of birth complications or having a newborn with a low birth weight (Gruber et al., 2013). A great deal of scholarship suggests that the time frame around childbirth and labor is stressful for the mothers (e.g., fears of pains, concerns for a baby's safety) (Lothian, 2009; Srisuthisak, 2009). It also is evident that maternal stress during labor and delivery can delay the onset of lactation and interfere with breastfeeding (Chen et al., 1998; Dewey et al., 2003; Tully & Ball, 2014).

History of Chinese Midwifery and Move to Modern Medicine in Twentieth-Century China

The history of Chinese midwifery can be divided into three phases: before 1929, an indigenous model; from 1929 to 2008, the establishment of a biomedical model; and after 2008, Chinese midwifery within nursing (Cheung, 2009; Harris et al., 2007). Tracking the changes that have occurred in relation to Chinese midwifery, we see that it has shifted from being an arena for the lay practitioner (also called *jieshengpo or chanpo* in Chinese) to professional staff—the modern midwife (also called *zhuchanshi* in Chinese).

In dynastic China, childbirth used to be a domestic affair attended to by women. Those women were mostly female family members or "birth grannies" (Cheung, 2009; Harris et al., 2007). Such birth grannies were married and had experienced childbirth. Traditional midwives were usually illiterate (Cheung, 2009). Like European or American midwives of the time, Chinese *jieshengpo* received their knowledge from other women who had experienced childbirth and labor as well as from their own experiences. Their responsibilities were focused on the birthing process. They usually came to the expectant mothers' home to assist the laboring process. *Jieshengpo* served a supporting role for women in labor in dynastic China until 1929.

Childbirth in China has changed dramatically since the early twentieth century. In 1929, the first biomedical midwifery school was established in Beijing. This was during the initial stages of the development of Western medicine in China (Buck, 1980; Cheung, 2009; Liu, 2005; Sidel & Sidel, 1974). Since then, many new midwives (*zhuchanshi* or birth helpers) have graduated from institutions like the First National Midwifery School, and most of them were young, unmarried, and trained in the disciplines of Western medicine. Trained midwives are different from the traditional *jieshengpo* in China, and these midwives are viewed as providing a relatively better sanitary birthing environment through the use of various medical instruments for pregnant women in labor (Harris et al., 2007; Phillips, 2007). From 1929 to 1949 (even before People's Republic China was established), the educated elite in China worshiped modernized science, technology, and medicine (Cheung, 2005). During the Cultural Revolution (1966–1972), midwifery education collapsed along with other higher education systems in China (Cheung, 2009). Chinese midwifery education was re-established at the end of 1972 and included the introduction of undergraduate education in nursing and postgraduate education (Cheung, 2009; Cheung et al., 2005; Smith & Tang, 2004).

Since 1979, under the leadership of Deng Xiaoping and through economic reforms, the Chinese healthcare system has had a profound shift. In order to improve health outcomes of women and children, the Chinese government has promoted a goal of moving all births into hospitals (The Central Committee of the Chinese Communist Party, 2002; Kelaher & Dollery, 2003). The shift of child birthing from private domestic places to the hospitals strengthens the power of the obstetrician and increased the marginalization of the midwife (Harris et al., 2007). For decades, midwifery did not have a clear professional location—it was not viewed as an obstetrics profession. For instance, in 1999, the Chinese Medical Practitioners' Law indicated that graduates in midwifery should not be able to work as medical physicians, and midwives were not qualified for advanced promotion (Butler, 2017; Cheung, 2009; Harris et al., 2007). In other words, the profession of midwifery was not supported by the government in the past. However, since 2008, the government has included the midwifery profession as part of the nursing profession (Cheung, 2009; Cheung & Mander, 2018). In order to work in a maternity hospital, a midwife has to pass the qualified nurse practitioner examination. Further, midwifery's higher education curriculum setting favors the nursing profession (Zhu et al. 2015). Nowadays, Chinese midwives' responsibilities consist of "preparing and maintaining the labor ward, monitoring women in labor, delivering babies, establishing early breast feeding, and record[ing] all medications and treatments for the birthing mothers, as well as assisting obstetricians with complex labors and other emergency obstetric care" (Harris et al., 2007, p. 208).

When the term "doula" was first introduced into China, its meanings were interpreted as "privately hired 'doula midwife'" (Cheung, 2009). According to Cheung et al. (2005, 2009), doula service—provision of companionship for birthing women and guiding women in labor—was welcomed by many families. In fact, this sort of support for childbirth is similar to the kind of support offered by the "old-wives" that Dalmiya and Alcoff (1993) write about. The doulas guide pregnant women by educating them about maternity and childbirth through an epistemology that privileges the processual. Thus, women's bodily birthing experiences are centered. It is essential to ask, *is it possible that these present-day Chinese doulas are recovering the role of "old-wives" or "birth grannies" through this revival of midwifery?*

Brief Introduction of Chinese Marketization Hospital

Since 1979, the reformed healthcare system in China has been an important component of the economic reforms resulting from the Open-Door Policy (Zheng, 2010; Yu, 2014; Ma et al., 2008, 2015). Because of the Open-Door Policy and the initial goal of national economic development, China integrated into the global market economy and the employed socialist market economy model (Ding, 2009). This transformation involved a change from a collective society of state-owned enterprises to new forms of private-enterprise ownership (Du, 2009; Ma et al., 2008). The healthcare system shifted from a government-centered/state-funded system to a market-oriented one (Blumenthal & Hsiao, 2005; Li et al., 2012). Within the economic reforms, the Chinese government liberalized private ownerships of many health facilities, particularly hospitals (Eggleston, 2010; Eggleston et al., 2009). A small city, Suqian in Jiangsu Province, pioneered in hospital reform by being the first city in China to sell government-run hospitals to private owners (Gu & Zhang, 2006; Harney & Jourdan, 2014). Suqian's bold decision originated from a reform measure passed by the State Council in 2000, which encouraged cooperation between and incorporation of various healthcare institutions (Duckett, 2012).

Along with the marketization of hospitals' ownership, the price of a liberalized system of hospital healthcare services was also promoted (Harris et al., 2007; Liu, 2004). One major and direct reason for hospital reform in China was insufficient government funding (Dyckerhoff & Wang, 2010; Ramesh et al., 2014). Local government provided the majority of government subsidy to public health, and they had a very strong incentive to shake off their financial burden (Gao, 2015; Wu et al., 2007). Likewise, hospital marketization was one of the most expedient ways to solve the government financial burden (Ramesh et al., 2014; Wu et al., 2007). However, the majority of China's medical facilities are still run by the central government and overseen by the Ministry of Health of the State Council (Fan, 2007; Harris et al., 2007). Therefore, contemporary Chinese hospitals operate under a combination of government management and private ownership.

WeCare Women's Maternity Hospital (hereafter WeCare WMH), the site of my field research, is a private maternity hospital under the leaderships of a city Public Health Bureau and a district/county Public Health Bureau.[2] Even though managed by government departments, the WeCare WMH could be viewed as a by-product of the marketization of hospital's ownership in China since the hospital makes its own management decisions and takes full responsibility for its own profits and losses (thus, it follows market economy logics).

Established around 2010, WeCare WMH is a private maternity hospital providing prenatal, childbirth, as well as postpartum habitation services for pregnant women. Importantly, WeCare WMH affiliates with Care Ambassador Hospital Group,[3] which provides various medical resources and networks. Since 2015, Care Ambassador Hospital Group has started partnerships with American International Childbirth Education Association, Transforming Maternity Care, and several American maternity hospitals/clinics. These collaborations focus on working together to improve the health and well-being of respective patient population, ongoing development of the maternity medical community, as well as developing expert-to-expert learning.

As part of laying the ground work for my research project in graduate school, I started an internship as a trainee of the public health service department at WeCare WMH in 2017.[4] With support and guidance from many faculty and staff at WeCare WMH, I successfully completed my 30-day trainee program. During my training, Childbirth Care[5]—an American childbirth education association—organized a

---

[2] WeCare Women's Maternity Hospital is located in a Chinese tier-one city. Therefore, it is under the leaderships of both city and district/county public health bureau offices.

[3] Care Ambassador Hospital Group is a national hospital group. I anonymize it in order to maintain confidentiality.

[4] WeCare WMH gave me lots of flexibilities for the internship. I was allowed to observe for most of the daily medial routine practices in the hospital.

[5] Childbirth Care is an American-based international childbirth education association. I anonymized the organization name in order to maintain the confidentiality.

seven-day childbirth education seminar at WeCare WMH. The seminar covered topics of ethics for childbirth educators, physiological process of birth in different stages, breastfeeding, postpartum care, emotional support, and advocacy for parents. I participated in the childbirth education seminar while also serving as a translator for parts of the seminar.[6] I also met more than 30 doulas, midwives, nurses, obstetricians, and childbirth educators who participated in the seminar and who came from different hospitals, organizations, or birth centers across the nation.

Back to 2017, I was still a doctoral student in graduate school. As a graduate student, I was extremely grateful to receive a training opportunity, in which I worked with and learnt from so many professional obstetric staff at WeCare WMH. Meanwhile, as a health communication researcher, my internship experience enabled me to closely observe and study with a unique group of healthcare workers within a Chinese hospital—maternal healthcare workers, including obstetricians, doulas, midwives, nurses, and childbirth educators. Importantly, I observed the nuance of doula care in China, in WeCare WMH, and among other maternity hospitals in China. Likewise, I recognized the scholarly and cultural importance of doulas and doula care as a unique group of healthcare workers. It is also important to point out WeCare WMH's specialties and distinctive features. It is a private maternity hospital associated with several international healthcare facilities; these features gave me an extraordinary opportunity to conduct research on Chinese maternity healthcare, maternal healthcare workers, and doulas.

Being a health communication researcher who received academic trainings from a school with a strong critical-cultural emphasis, I began to engage the research site with self-reflexivity. Believing in and utilizing reflexivity helped me to recognize that my personal experiences (interning at WeCare WMH) provide me considerable insights both for knowledge-information about others' lives and helped me to develop a capacity for insight, empathy, and attentive caring, particularly through interaction with participants (Alma & Smaling, 2006; Foss & Foss, 1994). By listening to stories from different obstetrics staff and maternity healthcare workers, I did not simply learn about what happened to them; I also came to understand their feelings, motivations for action, world views, and constructions of self. In particular, during the seven-day seminar with Childbirth Care Association, I talked with seminar participants about my research and heard many stories from their perspectives as mother doulas, hospital-based doulas, midwifery doulas, and obstetrics doulas. I was grateful that many of the seminar participants shared their interests and expressed their willingness to participate in my study. In fact, their interests and support provided an incentive for me to conduct my research.

I returned from WeCare WMH with clear direction and full of inspiration, appreciation, and a newfound understanding of how Chinese doulas, as an emerging group of maternity healthcare workers, can (re)define, conceptualize, and contribute to the complexity of respectful maternal healthcare in mainland China. Moreover,

---

[6] I served as a translator for the topics of emotional support, informational support, and shared decision-making process.

through the network I established in the internship, I had great opportunities to conduct interviews with doulas for this project and to hear women's voices from this unique group of maternal healthcare workers.

Context of Doula in China

Doula care is a relatively new maternity healthcare profession in mainland China. Dr. Defen Wang, an obstetrics staff member at Shanghai Maternity Health Hospital, introduced concepts of the doula and doula care into China in 1996 (Shu & Wang, 2002; Zheng et al., 2015). Dr. Wang translated the term "doula" as "*dao le*" in Chinese. However, the role of a doula and the ideas about doula care in pregnancy and labor took quite a few years to become known and accepted in Chinese clinical settings.

Prior to this book, I conducted a qualitative content analysis to analyze the discourse about doula profession, doula care and women in Chinese news coverage. A total of 76 doula-related news stories were reviewed and analyzed. Through the analysis, I found that the introduction of doulas as professional obstetric staff was highlighted by referencing women-centered maternal healthcare. This was seen in story headlines such as "*Women-Family-Centered Maternity with Doula Support*" and "*Doula Provides Support for Women in Labor.*" I also discovered that the introduction of doula care was often discussed in relation to cooperation with Western clinics, especially collaboration with American obstetric staffs. Interestingly, the *Six Healthy Birth Practices of Lamaze* were also an important theme that emerged alongside the international cooperation. One article titled "*Breathing Is Not Easy*" described a Lamaze training seminar that was held by Guangzhou Elizabeth Women's Hospital in 2013. Dr. Jeanette T. Crawshaw (the former chair of Lamaze and a professor from Texas Technology Nursing School) and several Chinese childbirth educators led the training. Training included guiding expectant mothers through several techniques in labor, including allowing labor to begin on its own, how to walk and change positions throughout labor, as well as bringing a doula for continuous support in labor.

Moreover, promotion of doula care in labor was another theme that emerged from the analysis. The articles "*Luoyang Maternity and Child Health Hospital Develops Doula Care in Labor*" and "*China Women's Development Foundation Promoted Doula Care Program in Chongqing*" suggested that doula care in labor is promoted and organized by officials in different cities in China. An article described the program of "*Doula Care in Chongqing*" was part of the Chongqing Women's Federation's development projects, alongside "*Reduce Breast Cancer and Ovarian Cancer*," "*Love in Action for Mothers*," and "*Elimination of Infant Anemia.*" It was important to point out that China Women's Development Foundation and Women's Federation in different cities were highly involved in the organization and promotion of doula care in labor. Besides Luoyang and Chongqing, Chinese officials also promoted doula support in labor in various hospitals in Shanghai, Guangzhou,

Baoji, Hangzhou, Lanzhou, Zhengzhou, Hohhot, and Qinhuangdao. The promotion program was a collaboration between Chinese Women's Development Foundation and local maternity health hospitals. As the Chinese maternal healthcare system suggested, the majority of local maternity and child health hospitals have been public hospitals. Besides public maternal hospitals, there is an increasing number of private maternal hospitals also adopting the model of "doula support in labor." As one article suggested, Hangzhou Aima Maternity Hospital and Gansu Maria Gynecology Hospital (located in Lanzhou) were two baby-friendly private hospitals that provided doula care for women in labor under the guideline of Hangzhou and Lanzhou Women's Federations, respectively.[7]

It was hard to retrieve precisely which actual date the term "doula" first appeared on the mainstream media. When I was in WeCare WMH, I had conversations (most of them were informal chats) with many pregnant women (more than 50 women) and discussed topics of doula and doula care with them. Some of them told me they had never heard the term or the concept until they visited WeCare WMH. Some of them informed me that they had heard about doulas, but they were not very sure about what a doula does. A small portion of the women I chatted with indicated that they understood the role of the doula and said they were thinking of hiring one for their own childbirth. In fact, my personal and scholar observation resonated the media discourse analysis on the doula profession and doula care. Although doula profession is not yet widespread in China, it is a promising profession with support and promotion from government, along with an increasing number of women who express interests and passion for it.

A growing number of doulas who have had pregnancy experiences (normally, they underwent childbirth themselves) and some relevant professional doula care trainings (e.g., seminars of childbirth from the Lamaze International, workshops of International Childbirth Education Certificate Association) are emerging in mainland China. In fact, Chinese doulas are obligated to register with some international official departments or organizations (e.g., DONA, Lamaze International, Childbirth Professional International, International Childbirth Education Association).

Some literature defines a doula as a "privately-hired labor delivery room midwife or nurse providing one-to-one care during labor" in Chinese cultural and medical contexts (Cheung et al., 2005; Zhai, 2005). The Chinese doula takes her lead from what she sees as the doula's purpose in a Chinese context and does not unthinkingly adopt definitions and structures handed down from Western doula associations. Chinese doulas are closely linked with Chinese midwifery in medical perception, and the cultural interpretation is linked to what local policy makers also observe (Cheung et al., 2005; Cheung et al., 2009).

Medical childbirth support, however, is mostly seen support through medical, herbal, and technological intervention. Yet, it is also true that, whether some medical structures in China acknowledge it or not, the provision of social, cultural, and

---

[7] The results of this analysis were originally published in the article *Chinese News Media Discourse of Doulas and Doula Care* (2018). I selected a few main findings from the 2018 article and presented here.

physical assistance is childbirth support (Basile, 2012; Iravani et al., 2015; Sheffey, 2017; Zauderer, 2009). Various cultures have childbirth support systems that address pregnant women's anxieties and concerns—the unknown factors that include fear, pain, and the possibility of death (Cohen & Mannarino, 2011; Haines et al., 2011). In particular, labor support—the provision of emotional, physical, and informational support—became a delimited role in the form of the doula (Hodnett et al., 2012; Torres, 2013).

The demand for doulas in China is increasing, and the rise in the use of doulas is thought to be due to the dissatisfaction with current institutional maternity healthcare. In fact, Chinese women are generally not provided the continuity of care and emotional support they want within the maternity system (Cheung et al., 2009; Gu et al., 2013; Homer et al., 2000; Raven et al., 2015). Thus, the increase in doulas and doula care during childbirth and pregnancy is both critical and demanded in Chinese cultural and medical contexts in order to respond to women's dissatisfaction with their support in labor.

The health movement of women working as doulas emerged in China during the late twentieth century, specifically in the context of the privatization of the hospital care systems in China. An increasing push toward globalization and the Open-Door Policy toward the West led to increased intercultural exchange and communication between China and the West. The idea of doula care and the doula profession was introduced to China within the socioeconomic context of larger policy shifts. Doula care was introduced mostly in private hospitals and has become a commodified service (Field observations, May 10, 2017). My central research questions for this project are in two clusters of questions:

Research question cluster 1: How does the larger context of policy shifts in the Chinese medical system toward privatization of medical care and toward Open-Door Policy shape the doula care system?

Research question cluster 2: Could doulas construct a supportive community and privilege women's autonomy and decision making individually in private hospital settings in order to empower women emotionally in the context of childbirth? How do the doulas negotiate this and other contradictions that emerge through their work?

Explanation of Method and Data: Interviewing

Interviewing is a useful and significant research method that qualitative researchers can "use to gain insight into the world of their respondents" (Hesse-Biber, 2006, p. 114). It is important to point out that interviewing as a qulitative research method has been used by scholars in various disciplines, including sociology, anthropology, nursing, and communication studies (see Kane Low et al., 2006; Lazarus, 1994; Stevens et al., 2011; Tetteh, 2018). Moreover, qualitative interviewing is one of the "preeminent methods in communication studies" since interviews "enable researchers to gather information about things or processes that cannot be observed effectively by other means" (Lindlof & Taylor, 2011, p.172-175). As an interpretive interviewer researching for a women-centered project, I am particularly interested in conducting research on "issues that [are] of concern to women's lives" (Hesse-Biber, 2006, p. 113). Thus, I focus on understanding the emergence of doula care and the role doulas play as a group of maternity healthcare workers in China. As doula care emerges as a viable profession for Chinese women, its nuances and contradictions can be revealed through a women-centered health communication lens. I therefore conducted interviews with professional doulas in China to collect data for this project.

At the start of this research project, I felt simultaneously wary and eager to use qualitative research methods. On one hand, most of the health communication researches conducted in communication studies have used various quantitative research methods while casting doubt on the use of qualitative methods. On the other hand, qualitative research methods offer both a very rich methodological literature and epistemology, which is well-suited to my research goal of exploring the practices of doulas as healthcare workers in China. However, I worked through my early self-doubt regarding methods and proceeded with the conviction that qualitative methods in this project were the most appropriate for my goals as a researcher. Using the method of interviews allowed me to provide the doulas (research participants) with opportunities to explore their motivations for being involved in doula work. The interviews mode therefore allowed me to examine and unpack how doula caregiving processes and techniques resonate with doulas' own beliefs and embodied experiences.

I am also influenced significantly by an interpretivist paradigm (in both theory and method). I suggest that using an embodied health communication research approach to study understudied health-related issues, such as Chinese doulas, doula care, the multiple roles of Chinese doulas in society, and the doulas' different identities, can lead to the production of valuable knowledge that will enhance an understanding of caring and health from the perspective of those affected (Jaggar, 2014).

To be eligible to participate in the research study, participants were required to meet specific criteria. Participants needed to have attended an initial doula education course (e.g., The International Childbirth Education Association workshop) during the past three or more months and needed to be currently practicing as doulas. This criterion ensured that participants had some experience in being doulas.

Sixteen Chinese doulas participated in this project. I recruited some of the interviewees from WeCare WMH, where I completed my internship. Some of the interviewees were recruited from the Childbirth Care Education seminar, which I participated in during my internship. My cohorts from the Childbirth Care Education seminar introduced me to many of their colleagues and friends, who also have worked as doulas and met the criteria to participate in this project. In other words, some of my interviewees were recruited through the networks I built with Chinese doulas and childbirth educators.

The median age for the 16 participants was 36.7 years, and their ages ranged from 27 to 64 years. Of the participants, 2 had some graduate education or master's degree, 13 had some college education or bachelor's degree, and 1 had a high school education. Seven participants went to medical schools or nursing schools and had worked (or were still working) as obstetricians, nurses, or midwives in the hospitals[8]. Nine of the participants did not receive any professional medical training before they dedicated their career to doula care. Three of the participants had worked as professional birth doulas for more than four years, seven of them had three years of experience working as doulas, four of them had one to two years of experience, and the rest two had less than one year of doula working experience. Ten of the participants described themselves as private doulas or called themselves "mother doulas." They worked for related doula organizations or were self-employed as mother doulas. The rest (N = 6) worked as hospital-based doulas or as obstetricians/midwives in a maternity hospital and had received professional doula care trainings as well as provided doula care for expectant mothers in laboring. Fifteen participants were married, one participant was divorced, and all of them were heterosexual. Only one participant did not have childbirth experience herself, and the rest of them had at least one childbirth experience. Seven of the participants worked and lived, at the time of interview, in one of China's four municipalities (Beijing, Shanghai, Tianjin, and Chongqing). Four of the participants currently worked and lived in one of the capital cities of China's provinces (e.g., Guangzhou, Guangdong Province; Hangzhou, Zhejing Province; Zhengzhou, capital of Henan Province, etc.). The rest (N = 5) lived and worked in the non-capital cities (e.g., Zhuhai in Guangzhou Province, Quanzhou in Fujian Province, Luoyang in Henan Province). (See complete demographic information in Table 1.1).

I used pseudonyms for all participants in order to maintain confidentiality. According to their self-descriptions, most of the participants have worked in multiple professions as childbirth health workers, including doulas, childbirth educators, lactation consultants, obstetricians, and midwives. (See details about each doula's childbirth experience, working statuses, as well as a short biography in the following paragraphs).[9]

Ai Bei: Ai Bei has worked as a midwife for more than 35 years. She used to work in a public maternity hospital. After she officially retired several years ago, she started to work in private maternity hospitals. In 2015, Ai Bei began training in doula care when the hospital she worked for coordinated related seminars. She is in her 60s and is married. She has an associate degree in nursing.

He Pei: He Pei described herself as an obstetrician, lactation consultant, doula, and childbirth educator. She used to work as an obstetrician in a public hospital. About three years ago, she switched her work from clinical obstetrician to childbirth educator and researcher in the hospital. He Pei is in her 40s. She graduated from a

---

[8] In China, universities are able to provide bachelor's and master's degrees in nursing, medicine, and related medical fields. Thus, some of the participants can hold bachelor's degrees in medicine and work as obstetrician/physician in one hospital.

[9] I listed participants' names based on the alphabetic orders of their pseudonyms' family names. In Chinese culture, the order of a person's name is family name and then given time. It is in a different order from an American name.

medical school with a master's degree. She is married with one child. Currently, He Pei works at a public hospital in a capital city as a childbirth educator and research faculty.

Huang Ru: Huang Ru described herself as a mother doula and lactation consultant. Three years ago, she started to learn about doula care and hydrotherapy during labor (she was pregnant at the time). Huang Ru graduated from college with an education major. Before she started to work as a doula, Huang worked as a preschool teacher. Huang divorced her husband in 2016.

Jiang Min: Jiang Min worked for an international business company for a decade. After she had her child, she dedicated her career to breastfeeding and childbirth education. She owns her own business as a lactation consultant and doula. She participated in several childbirth education seminars held by some related childbirth/doula care organizations. She is in her 30s and married.

Jian Ning: Jian Ning described herself as a mother doula, lactation consultant, and childbirth educator. She owns her own business as a doula and lactation consultant. Jian Ning graduated from college with a business major. She received doula training and related childbirth education about three years ago. She is married with two children. Jian Ning is in her 30s.

Lin Jing: Lin Jing owns her own business as a mother doula and lactation consultant. She started her business in early 2016. Lin Jing used to be a professional sport athlete and comes from a non-medical background. Lin Jing is in her late 20s and is married with two children.

Liu Ying: Liu Ying used to work as an obstetrician for a government-based maternal hospital. She had her child in early 2016. Then, Liu started to work as a childbirth educator and researcher in the hospital's public health department. She explained that the reason she changed her position was because of her child. She is in her mid-30s and married.

Ming Jing: Ming Jing had worked as a nurse for more than 30 years. She started to receive doula and related childbirth training in early 2016. She works as a childbirth educator for a private hospital, which mainly focuses on maternal healthcare education. She is in her early 60s and married with one child.

Qin Nan: Qin Nan graduated from a nationally ranked university with a bachelor's degree in general medicine. After she graduated, she worked for a government-based hospital for several years. Since 2010, she has been involved with different doulas and doula care promotion programs across the nation. Qin Nan works for a nationwide doula profession organization. She has worked closely with several national-/regional-related official public health or women's health organizations. Qin Nan is married with one child.

Shen Yu: Shen Yu has worked as a hospital-based doula since early 2016. She graduated from a college with a business major. She is in her 30s and is married with one child. She delivered the baby in a private hospital with professional doula support. Since then, she has learned more about doula care and gentle birth. She has participated in several doula care and childbirth trainings.

Su Yi: Su Yi used to work as an obstetrician for a government-based maternal hospital. She has worked the last eight years in a private maternal hospital. Su Yi received a bachelor's degree from a medical school focusing on obstetrics. She began related doula care training in early 2016. She is married with no children.

Wang Wei: Wang Wei has worked as a nurse in a government-based hospital for several years and is a licensed practical nurse. She described herself as a nurse, lactation consultant, and doula. Initially, Wang Wei started to learn about breastfeeding and lactation after delivering her baby. Now, she participates in different doula care training programs. She is married with one son and has graduated from a nationally ranked medical school with a nursing degree. She is in her 30s.

Xue Li: Xue Li described herself as a doula and lactation consultant. She has a non-medical education background and started to work as a lactation consultant about four years ago. She started to work as a doula after participating in several doula care training programs. She is married with one child. Xue Li is in her 30s.

Xue Meimei: Xue Meimei described herself as a mother doula and lactation consultant. She came from a non-medical education background and started to work in childbirth education about four years ago. She is in her 30s and is married with one child.

Yue Le: Yue Le has worked as a midwife for 10 years. She worked for a public hospital for seven years before switching to a private maternal hospital. She began doula care and childbirth-related training about a couple of years ago. She is married with one child.

Zeng Rui: Zeng Rui owns her own business as a doula, lactation consultant, and childbirth educator. She graduated from college with a business major and worked for several business management companies for years. On behalf of her business, Zeng Rui has coordinated with several childbirth associations for many childbirth/women's health-related seminars and activities. She is in her 30s and is married with one child. Zeng Rui lives in a non-capital city.

Semi-structured, interviews ranged in length from 40 to 75 min. Interviews were conducted face-to-face or through a voice/video call using the Chinese messaging app WeChat (also recognized as a social media app). All interviews were conducted in Chinese, and the transcriptions were also analyzed in Chinese.

Inspired by previous qualitative women's health projects (Tetteh, 2018; Dwyer, 2012; Hanasono, 2018), I analyzed the data by utilizing grounded theory (Charmaz, 2014; Strauss & Corbin, 1990). Grounded theory involves initial coding where the researcher interacts with the data to understand what is happening and focused coding where he/she develops initial codes to synthesize and organize the data as well as to develop theory (Corbin & Strauss, 1990; Morse & Field, 1995; Strauss & Corbin, 1990). Likewise, grounded theory allows themes to emerge out of the data. After I transcribed the interviews, I familiarized myself with the transcripts by reading and re-reading them with the intent of allowing major themes to emerge naturally. Line-by-line coding actions helped me to separate the data into categories and to identity key concepts (Charmaz, 2014; Glaser & Strauss, 1967).

Health Communication, Positionality, and Reflexivity

Health communication includes various forms of communication in everyday contexts of healthcare and in the healthcare industry. Lindlof and Taylor (2011) define health communication as "a subfield that represents a distinctive genre of applied research that was founded by post positivist scholars of interpersonal and mass communication" (p. 19). They also refer to health communication as traditionally assisting healthcare professionals in identifying and overcoming perceived communication problems that affect public health as well as the delivery of health services (Lindlof & Taylor, 2011). Lindlof and Taylor also express their concerns about the status quo of health communication research methods. They state that without looking at various research methods health communication studies will continue to maintain the "hierarchical authority of medical professionals over patients" (p. 19). Failure to examine the role of power and of socially constructed discourse in healthcare settings has resulted in important gaps in health communication scholarship. The lack of a critical-cultural perspective in examining communication among health caregivers, for instance, limits the research inquiry in the field of health communication.

The critique of status quo health communication research offers support to the argument that health communication needs to begin involving more critical-cultural approaches in order to understand how unequal power relations impact the quality of healthcare. There is also a need to examine how power is exercised and how the body is disciplined, surveilled, trained, and controlled (Foucault, 1979). In the article *Toward the Development of Critical Health Communication Praxis*, Deborah Lupton (1994) discusses the problems of power, structure, and control in healthcare settings. Works by health communication scholars such as Lupton, Dutta, and Basu have raised concerns around issues of power, discipline, and surveillance and have provided opportunities for others to embrace theoretical and methodological shifts in order to include a critical-cultural perspective and to develop a cultural-centered approach (Dutta, 2010; Dutta & Basu, 2008). However, critical research approaches to the study of health campaigns and health discourse have a much older history. Development communication scholars, such as Phyllis Dako-Gyeke et al. (2015), have conducted research through the use of critical communication research methods in their works in the context of Ghana. Further, scholars such as Paula Triechler (2012) have been researching AIDS through a critical feminist lens since the 1980s. Such work as hers predates even the current move in health communication toward critical and cultural research methods. My work draws on these trends in critical communication research methods being used in the study of health communication and contributes to the increasing body of work that comes under the heading of "critical health communication."

The goal of critical health communication is to provide an alternative entry point for theorizing and practicing health communication by highlighting the absences and/or silences in current positivist health communication and by presenting voices of the marginalized groups through engagement in the dialogue (Airhihenbuwa,

1995; Dutta, 2007; Dutta-Bergman, 2004a, b, 2005). There is a growing number of critical communication scholars (e.g., Amber Basu, Heather Zoller, Laura Ellingson, Radhika Gajjala, Marina Levina) starting to explore issues of domination and power in the field of health communication.

Annandale (2003) suggests that "health has been a crucial vehicle for the development of feminist theory" (p. 4). Therefore, many critical health scholars have problematized the contemporary medicalization of women's bodies, which institutionally press for medical intervention and maintain power over women, especially through women's reproductive agency and the power dynamics of medical knowledge (Clarke, 1998; Brubaker & Dillaway, 2009; Chikovore, 2004; Martin, 2001; Sherwin, 1998). In order to "demystify and democratize" medical knowledge and to empower women, feminist health researchers have advocated that women should establish women-centered health organizations as well as birth centers (Morgan, 1998, p, 113; Turshen, 2007).

The One-Child Policy was implemented in China in 1979. Thus, within a framework of economic development, Chinese women of childbearing age were all affected by the nationwide One-Child Policy (Milwertz, 1997). The policy was supposed to curtail unprecedented population growth so that overpopulation would not interrupt economic growth, which was a key focus of the government beginning with the Open-Door Policy[10] in the late 1970s (Zhang, 2008).

From 1979 to 2015, the One-Child Policy brought about a shortage of younger relatives to care for an aging population. The nation has also faced a labor shortage. The Chinese National Health and Family Planning Commission states that "abolishing the one-child policy would increase labor supply and ease pressures from an aging population" (Buckley, 2015). Therefore, China shifted from the One-Child Policy to the Second-Child Policy by the end of 2015 in order to support "sustained and healthy economic development" (Zraick, 2015). When the One-Child Policy was ended in 2015, it announced that all legally married couples were permitted to have a second child in their families. In 2016, China had 140 million women of childbearing age who had already raised a child; now, they were expected to have a second child (Zeng & Hesketh, 2016). Chinese women are, therefore, currently allowed to have two children. As a result of the policy, it fulfilled the demand for labor, which has been on a decrease, as well as increased expectations on women to have a second child as this developed into a cultural nation.

For the past few years, my research has been focused on Chinese women's bodies, women's reproductive rights, and maternity healthcare in general. Theoretical frameworks and methodological interventions made by several outstanding researchers of communication serve as a guide for me (see Yahui Zhang, 2008; Radhika Gajjala, 2002; Paula Triechler, 1990). When I first began to work with maternal healthcare workers (e.g., doulas, midwives, obstetricians, nurses, childbirth educators) in China, I struggled with questions about how I could juggle my

---

[10] The Open-Door Policy of the People's Republic of China was initiated in 1979. The Chinese leadership has attached to the goals of strengthening the country's economic potential and moving toward industrialization and urbanization (Liu, 2011; Bohnet et al., 1993).

roles as a health communication researcher and a woman, while also being myself an advocate for the doula profession. Therefore, the writing process of this project is both an exercise in self-comprehension and an exploration and in-depth understanding of doula care as an emerging maternal healthcare profession.

This project is also inspired by previous studies on women's health (e.g., reproductive rights, ovarian cancers, miscarriage, and doulas) in various cultural and medical contexts (e.g., American, Canadian, Australian, Chinese, Ghanaian), (Dwyer, 2012; Basile, 2012; Fulton, 2011; Hunter & Hurst, 2016; Hanasono, 2018; Ding et al., 2018; Jiang, 2018; Tetteh, 2017). The overall project explores the Chinese doulas' identity construction and doula care practice.

I wrote this project from the subject position of a Chinese woman born and raised in China and also as someone who has not herself actually experienced childbirth. It is important to point out that I recognize my personal and scholarly standpoints regarding "power and authority over the interview situation" (Hesse-Biber, 2006, p.114). In other words, I understand that I speak from a socially and culturally privileged location because of my higher education experience in the United States. Many of my urban Chinese women counterparts, who are situated in a different setting geographically, materially, and culturally, have not had access to the same social, cultural, and educational opportunities that I have. Also, I grew up in a time period when China started to engage in economic and healthcare reforms and became integrated into the global system. My positionality and perspectives are clearly influenced by my biography, experience, and knowledge.

Personal experience in research is valuable in that it is beneficial not only to the scholar but also to the participants. Sometimes, scholars may argue about whether research through women's experience could be beneficial to their lives, but feminist scholars counter such an argument. They note that, when people listen to women's (or men's) "real" lives and focus on their "real" stories, then research can contribute to the improvement of participants' lives by encouraging them to think critically about their lives.

Importantly, bringing my own experiences as a Chinese woman into the project makes it possible for me to engage in reflexivity. As Hesse-Biber (2007) argues, "Reflexivity, at one level, is a self-critical action whereby the researcher finds that the world is mediated by the self—what can be known can only be known through oneself, one's lived experience, and one's biography" (p. 496). Being reflexive is significant for my project because I have not experienced pregnancy and labor first-hand. All the knowledge I have about pregnancy and childbirth is from the secondary sources including books, newspapers, and research articles, which are sources that sometimes give limited representations of the experiences (Stacey, 1997).

Moreover, I acknowledge that my identity as a researcher (e.g., I come from different sociocultural backgrounds than many participants) and as an outsider to Chinese doulas might have impacted how the women related to me and how they chose to share their experiences. These differences could be advantageous in that I asked questions about topics that participants and insiders would have taken for granted, but the differences also presented some challenges (Blythe et al., 2013).

The purpose of engaging in the reflexivity is to place Chinese doulas' experiences and their knowledge into the "center of social inquiry" (Chiseri-Strater, 1996; Jessor & Colby, 1996) and to better inform my interpretation of their experiences.

Further, the methods of data collection (i.e., face-to-face interviews, WeChat interviews) might have affected how Chinese women presented their narratives and how I interpreted their representation of their experiences. For instance, lack of physical contact in a WeChat interview might have enhanced or inhibited a woman's comfort level to share their experiences.

By the time I have finished my internship and interviews with participants, I am enlightened about women's pregnancy and childbirth as well as the hard and significant work that doulas and maternity healthcare workers perform. Through the time I participated in the Childbirth Care Education seminar, the days and nights I worked with many obstetrics staff in WeCare WMH, as well as the stories I heard about Chinese women's pregnancy and laboring, I have been motivated, inspired, and enlightened. All these gave me a new understanding and appreciation for pregnant women (birthing mothers), doulas, midwives, nurses, obstetricians, childbirth educators, along with Chinese women in general.

Significance of the Study

A large number of health communication studies have examined problems intrinsic to the organizational and interpersonal practice of health, such as the application of technology in the treatment of diverse populations and in doctor–patient relationships (see Azad, 2017; Sun et al., 2017; Zhou et al., 2017). This project contributes to scholarship about women's health as well as Chinese women's pregnancy and childbirth in general. Importantly, this project is focusing on doulas—a nuanced group of maternal healthcare workers—and the doula care profession in China.

As a health communication researcher, I focus my attention on women's relationships with their bodies and on women's experiences of choice, and access to health and reproductive services. Likewise, doula care in childbirth is important to the health communication research agenda because it is concerned with questions about who has access to respectful maternal healthcare information and support, as well as how information about childbirth is (re)presented and communicated.

As a person who grew up in China, my own experiences also inform my research on how Chinese society is able to mobilize different discourses to move forward maternity healthcare policies. Moreover, this project focuses on how Chinese obstetrics staff (including doulas, midwives, nurses, obstetricians, health workers, and childbirth educators) construct a discourse about the themes and have dialogues that characterize the contemporary Chinese medical environment, particularly in terms of maternal healthcare and reproductive rights.

This project, therefore, is not only dedicated to doulas and obstetrics staff in China, but to women in general. Furthermore, this study is for scholars, researchers, and health practitioners who are interested in issues related to women, maternity, and healthcare research in China. For practitioners and clinicians, especially doulas, midwives, and obstetricians, I would like to foreground their voice. In addition, this project offers an alternative and health communication lens to look at maternal healthcare and childbirth in the context of contemporary Chinese healthcare.

In this project, I examine how Chinese doulas construct multiple identities in terms of serving as lactation consultants, child care providers, and child care educators for women during pregnancy and childbirth. Chinese doulas develop a close relationship with pregnant women as sisters and families. Importantly, Chinese doulas are a female healthcare worker group, and their population is diverse and unique in terms of women's different and various backgrounds. Doula support not only has been explored in labor and childbirth, but also has been introduced to women in pregnancy and women in general as a notion of respectful maternal healthcare. The provision of doulas' support to Chinese pregnant women and expectant mothers constructs a space outside of mainstream Chinese medical and hospital-based healthcare sittings.

Overview of the Book

In the following chapters, I draw from relevant literature to analyze and discuss the research findings. I explore the discourse of the doula profession and doula care in Chinese maternity healthcare. I also examine the topics of natural delivery and usage of epidural analgesic for labor pain management alongside the doulas' interest in respecting Chinese women's choice, the construction of sisterhood, and the tensions and conflicts between professional doulas and obstetricians and midwives.

From Chaps. 2, 3, 4, 5 and 6, I provide a comprehensive analysis and discussion of the many facets of Chinese doulas and doula care, particularly the societal factors and political policies that influence maternal healthcare in China. These chapters are drawn from the main themes that emerged in the interviews. Specific purposes and objectives are to identify how Chinese doulas see their roles, provide insights into what the doula care perspective contributes to Chinese maternal healthcare, define the health and relational implications of the related perceptions, and increase a public understanding of Chinese doulas in general.

In the last chapter, I weave the gist of my project's analysis and conclusions with my family stories and scholarly reflection on the entire project. The goal of this research is to unravel the workings of power structures and to invite continued discussion and analysis that can inform strategies for actions. There are many possibilities for continued research on women's childbirth experiences and for the working experiences of doulas and related professional childbirth workers in China. Thus, my project is a starting point for future interdisciplinary projects.

References

Airhihenbuwa, C. O. (1995). *Health and culture: Beyond the Western paradigm.* Sage.

Alma, H., & Smaling, A. (2006). The meaning of empathy and imagination in health care and health studies. *International Journal of Qualitative Studies on Health and Wellbeing, 1*(4), 195–211. https://doi.org/10.1080/17482620600789438

Amram, N. L., Klein, M. C., Mok, H., Simkin, P., Lindstrom, K., & Grant, J. (2014). How birth doulas help clients adapt to changes in circumstances, clinical care, and client preferences during labor. *The Journal of Perinatal Education, 23*(2), 96–103. https://doi.org/10.1891/1058-1243.23.2.96

Annandale, E. (2003). *Feminist theory and the sociology of health and illness.* Routledge.

Azad, K. A. K. (2017). Media and doctor-patient relationship. *Journal of Medicine, 18*(1), 1. https://doi.org/10.3329/jom.v18i1.31161

Bäckström, C., & Hertfelt Wahn, E. (2011). Support during labour: first-time fathers' descriptions of requested and received support during the birth of their child. *Midwifery, 27*(1), 67–73. https://doi.org/10.1016/j.midw.2009.07.001

Basile, M. R. (2012). *Reproductive justice and childbirth reform: Doulas as agents of social change* (Doctoral Dissertation). University of Iowa, IA. Retrieved from ProQuest.

Blumenthal, D., & Hsiao, W. (2005). Privatization and its discontents—The evolving Chinese health care system. *New England Journal of Medicine, 353*(11), 1165–1170.

Blythe, S., Wükes, L., Jackson, D., & Halcomb, E. (2013). The challenges of being an insider in storytelling research. *Nurse Researcher, 21*(1), 8–13. https://doi.org/10.7748/nr2013.09.21.1.8.e333

Bohnet, A., Hong, Z. & Müller, F. (1993). China's open-door policy and its significance for transformation of the economic system. *Intereconomics, 28*, 191–197. https://doi.org/10.1007/BF02926200

Brubaker, S. J., & Dillaway, H. E. (2009). Medicalization, natural childbirth and birthing experiences. *Sociology Compass, 3*(1), 31–48. https://doi.org/10.1111/j.1751-9020.2008.00183.x

Buck, P. (1980). *American science and modern China, 1876-1936.* Cambridge University Press.

Buckley, C. (2015, October 30). China ends one-child policy, allowing families two children. *The New York Times.* Retrieved from https://www.nytimes.com/2015/10/30/world/asia/china-end-one-child-policy.html

Butler, J. (2017). Maternity services in china and professional identity of the midwife. *British Journal of Midwifery, 25*(6), 396–400. https://doi.org/10.12968/bjom.2017.25.6.396

Campbell, D. A., Lake, M. F., Falk, M., & Backstrand, J. R. (2006). A randomized control trial of continuous support in labor by a lay doula. *Journal of Obstetric, Gynecologic, & Neonatal Nursing., 35*, 456–464.

Charmaz, K. (2014). Grounded theory in global perspective: Reviews by international researchers. *Qualitative Inquiry, 20*(9), 1074–1084. https://doi.org/10.1177/1077800414545235

Chen, D., Nommsen-Rivers, L., Dewey, K., & Lonnerdal, B. (1998). Stress during labor and delivery and early lactation performance. *American Journal of Clinical Nutrition, 68*(2), 335–344.

Cheung, N. F. (2009). Chinese midwifery: the history and modernity. *Midwifery, 25*(3), 228–241.

Cheung, N. F., & Mander, R. (2018). *Midwifery in China.* Routledge. https://doi.org/10.4324/9781351124522

Cheung, N. F., Mander, R., & Cheng, L. (2005). The 'doula-midwives' in Shanghai. *Evidence Based Midwifery, 3*(2), 73–80.

Cheung, N. F., Mander, R., Wang, X., Fu, W., & Zhu, J. (2009). Chinese midwives' views on a proposed midwife-led normal birth unit. *Midwifery, 25*(6), 744–755. https://doi.org/10.1016/j.midw.2009.03.008

Chiseri-Strater, E. (1996). Turning in upon ourselves: Positionality, subjectivity, and reflexivity in case study and ethnographic research. In P. Mortensen & G. E. Kirsch (Eds.), *Ethics and representation in qualitative studies of literacy* (pp. 115–133). National Council of Teachers of English (NCTE).

Clarke, A. (1998). *Disciplining reproduction: Modernity, American life sciences, and "The Problems of Sex"*. University of California Press.

Chikovore, J. (2004). Gender power dynamics in sexual and reproductive health: A qualitative study in Chiredzi district, Zimbabwe (Publication No. 401018:2004) [Doctoral dissertation, Umeå University]. Retrieved from ProQuest.

Chor, J., Goyal, V., Roston, A., Keith, L., & Patel, A. (2012). Doulas as facilitators: The expanded role of doulas into abortion care. *Journal of Family Planning and Reproductive Health Care, 38*(2), 123–124. https://doi.org/10.1136/jfprhc-2011-100278

Cohen, J. A., & Mannarino, A. P. (2011). Supporting children with traumatic grief: What educators need to know. *School Psychology International, 32*(2), 117–131. https://doi.org/10.1177/0143034311400827

Corbin, J. M., & Strauss, A. (1990). Grounded theory research: Procedures, canons, and evaluative criteria. *Qualitative Sociology, 13*(1), 3–21.

Dahlen, H. G., Jackson, M., & Stevens, J. (2011). Homebirth, freebirth and doulas: Casualty and consequences of a broken maternity system. *Women and Birth, 24*(1), 47–50. https://doi.org/10.1016/j.wombi.2010.11.002

Dako-Gyeke, M., Dako-Gyeke, P., & Asampong, E. (2015). Experiences of stigmatization and discrimination in accessing health services: Voices of persons living with HIV in Ghana. *Social Work in Health Care, 54*(3), 269–285. https://doi.org/10.1080/00981389.2015.1005268

Dalmiya, V., & Alcoff, L. (1993). Are "old wives' tales" justified? In L. Alcoff & E. Potter (Eds.), *Feminist Epistemology* (pp. 217–244). Routledge.

Davis-Floyd, R. E. (2004). *Birth as an American rite of passage: With a new preface*. University of California Press. https://doi.org/10.1525/j.ctt1pndwn

Dewey, K. G., Nommsen-Rivers, L. A., Heinig, M. J., & Cohen, R. J. (2003). Risk factors for suboptimal infant breastfeeding behavior, delayed onset of lactation, and excess neonatal weight loss. *Pediatrics, 112*, 607–619.

Ding, X. (2009). The Socialist Market Economy: China and the World. *China: Socialism, Capitalism, Market: Why Not? Where Next?, 73*(2), 235–241.

Ding, G., Tian, Y., Yu, J., & Vinturache, A. (2018). Cultural postpartum practices of 'doing the month' in China. *Perspectives in Public Health, 138*(3), 147–149. https://doi.org/10.1177/1757913918763285

DONA International, (n.d.). About DONA International. Retrieved November 5, 2021 from https://www.dona.org/the-dona-advantage/about/

Du, J. (2009). Economic reforms and health insurance in China. *Social Science & Medicine, 69*(3), 387–395. https://doi.org/10.1016/j.socscimed.2009.05.014

Duckett, J. (2012). *The Chinese state's retreat from health: Policy and the politics of retrenchment*. Routledge. https://doi.org/10.4324/9780203840726

Dundek, L. H. (2006). Establishment of a Somali doula program at a large metropolitan hospital. *The Journal of Perinatal & Neonatal Nursing, 20*(2), 128–137.

Dutta, M. J. (2007). *Communicating Health: A culture-centered approach* (1st ed.). Polity Press.

Dutta, M. J. (2010). The critical cultural turn in health communication: Reflexivity, solidarity, and praxis. *Health Communication, 25*(6-7), 534–539.

Dutta, M. J., & Basu, A. (2008). Meanings of health: Interrogating structure and culture. *Health communication, 23*(6), 560–572.

Dutta-Bergman, M. J. (2004a). Primary sources of health information: Comparisons in the domain of health attitudes, health cognitions, and health behaviors. *Health Communication, 16*(3), 273–288.

Dutta-Bergman, M. J. (2004b). The unheard voices of Santalis: Communicating about health from the margins of India. *Communication Theory, 14*(3), 237–263.

Dutta-Bergman, M. J. (2005). Theory and practice in health communication campaigns: A critical interrogation. *Health Communication, 18*(2), 103–122.

Dwyer, J. (2012). *Continuums of reproductive choice: Theorizing doula care* (Doctoral Dissertation). Carleton University, Ottawa, Canada. Retrieved from ProQuest.

Dyckerhoff, C. S., & Wang, J. (2010). China's health care reforms. *Health International,* *10*(November), 55–67. Retrieved from https://www.mckinsey.com/~/media/mckinsey/dot-com/client_service/healthcare%20systems%20and%20services/health%20international/hi10_china_healthcare_reform.ashx

Eggleston, K. (2010). 'Kan Bing Nan, Kan Bing Gui': Challenges for China's healthcare system thirty years into reform. *Growing Pains: Tensions and Opportunities in China's Transformation.* Stanford, CA: Walter H. Shorenstein Asia–Pacific Research Center.

Eggleston, K., Shen, Y., Lu, M., Li, C., Wang, J., Yang, Z., & Zhang, J. (2009). Soft budget constraints in china: Evidence from the Guangdong hospital industry. *International Journal of Health Care Finance and Economics, 9*(2), 233–242. https://doi.org/10.1007/s10754-0099067-1

Fan, R. (2007). Corrupt practices in Chinese medical care: The root in public policies and a call for Confucian-market approach. *Kennedy Institute of Ethics Journal, 17*(2), 111–131. https://doi.org/10.1353/ken.2007.0012

Foss, K. A., & Foss, S. K. (1994). Personal experience as evidence in feminist scholarship. *Western Journal of Communication, 58*(1), 39–43. https://doi.org/10.1080/10570319409374482

Foucault, M. (1979). *Discipline and punish: The birth of the prison* (Trans. from French by Alan Sheridan). New York: Vintage Books.

Fulton, J. M. (2011). *Doula supported childbirth: An exploration of maternal sensitivity, self- efficacy, responsivity, and parental attunement* (Doctoral Dissertation). University of California, Davis, CA. Retrieved from ProQuest.

Gajjala, R. (2002). An interrupted Postcolonial/Feminist cyberethnography: Complicity and resistance in the "cyberfield". *Feminist Media Studies, 2*(2), 177–193. https://doi.org/10.1080/14680770220150854

Gao, J. (2015). *Corporate governance in hospital: Case of public hospital corporate governance structure reform in China* (Doctoral dissertation). Retrieved from https://repositorio.iscte-iul.pt/bitstream/10071/11555/1/GAOJIE-Dissertation.pdf

Gentry, Q. M., Nolte, K. M., Gonzalez, A., Pearson, M., & Ivey, S. (2010). "Going beyond the call of doula": A grounded theory analysis of the diverse roles community-based doulas play in the lives of pregnant and parenting adolescent mothers. *The Journal of Perinatal Education, 19*(4), 24–40. https://doi.org/10.1624/105812410X530910

Gilliland, A. L. (2002). Beyond holding hands: The modern role of the professional doula. *Journal of Obstetric, Gynecologic & Neonatal Nursing, 31*(6), 762–769. https://doi.org/10.1177/0884217502239215

Glaser, B., & Strauss, A. (1967). The discovery of grounded theory. *London: Weidenfeld and Nicholson, 24*(25), 288–304.

Gruber, K. J., Cupito, S. H., & Dobson, C. F. (2013). Impact of doulas on healthy birth outcomes. *The Journal of Perinatal Education, 22*(1), 49–58. https://doi.org/10.1891/1058-1243.22.1.49

Gu, E., & Zhang, J. (2006). Health care regime change in urban china: Unmanaged marketization and reluctant privatization. *Pacific Affairs, 79*(1), 49–71.

Gu, C., Wu, X., Ding, Y., Zhu, X., & Zhang, Z. (2013). The effectiveness of a Chinese midwives' antenatal clinic service on childbirth outcomes for primipare: A randomized controlled trial. *International Journal of Nursing Studies, 50*(12), 1689–1697. https://doi.org/10.1016/j.ijnurstu.2013.05.001

Haines, H., Pallant, J. F., Karlström, A., & Hildingsson, I. (2011). Cross-cultural comparison of levels of childbirth-related fear in an Australian and Swedish sample. *Midwifery, 27*(4), 560–567. https://doi.org/10.1016/j.midw.2010.05.004

Hanasono, L. (2018, April 15). *The M-word: Shattering the Silence about Miscarriage.* [Video file]. Retrieved from https://www.youtube.com/watch?v=cwNXxErzoQ8&feature=youtu.be

Harney, A., & Jourdan, A., (2014, October 6) Dearth of doctors drags on china private health-care drive. *Reuters, World News.* Retrieved from https://www.reuters.com/article/us-china-healthcare-private/dearth-of-doctors-drags-on-china-private-healthcare-drive-idUSKCN0HV21T20141006

Harris, A., Belton, S., Barclay, L., & Fenwick, J. (2007). Midwives in China: 'jie sheng po' to 'zhu chan shi'. *Midwifery, 25*(2), 203–212. https://doi.org/10.1016/j.midw.2007.01.015

He, M. (2011). Doulas Going Dutch: The Role of Professional Labor Support in the Netherlands. *Independent Study Project (ISP) Collection*, Paper 1153. Retrieved from http://digitalcollections.sit.edu/isp_collection/1153

Hesse-Biber, S. (2006). The practice of feminist in-depth interviewing. In *The practice of qualitative interviewing* (pp. 111–148). Sage.

Hesse-Biber, S. (2007). *Handbook of feminist research: Theory and praxis*. Sage.

Hodnett, E. D., Gates, S., Hofmeyr, G. J., & Sakala, C. (2007). Continuous support for women during childbirth. *Cochrane Database of Systematic Reviews, 7*. Retrieved from http://www.european-doula-network.org/media/studies/Chocrane%20continuous%20support.pdf

Hodnett, E. D., Gates, S., Hofmeyr, G. J., Sakala, C., & Weston, J. (2012). Continuous support for women during childbirth. *Cochrane Database System Review, 10*. Retrieved from https://www.ncbi.nlm.nih.gov/pmc/articles/PMC4175537/

Homer, C., Davis, G., & Brodie, P. (2000). What do women feel about community-based antenatal care? *Australian and New Zealand Journal of Public Health, 24*(6), 590–595.

Hunter, C. A., & Hurst, A. (2016). *Understanding doulas and childbirth: Women, love, and advocacy*. Palgrave Macmillan. https://doi.org/10.1057/978-1-137-48536-6

Iravani, M., Zarean, E., Janghorbani, M., & Bahrami, M. (2015). Women's needs and expectations during normal labor and delivery. *Journal of Education and Health Promotion, 4*(6). https://doi.org/10.4103/2277-9531.151885

Jaggar, A. M. (2014). Introduction: The project of feminist methodology. In A. M. Jaggar (Ed.), *Just methods: An interdisciplinary feminist reader (vii-xiii)*. Paradigm Publishers.

Jessor, R., & Colby, A. (1996). In R. A. Shweder (Ed.), *Ethnography and human development: Context and meaning in social inquiry*. University of Chicago Press.

Jiang, W. (2018). *How do Chinese college students seek information to prevent unwanted pregnancy? A study of online information seeking for contraception* [Unpublished doctoral dissertation]. Bowling Green State University.

Kane Low, L., Moffat, A., & Brennan, P. (2006). Doulas as community health workers: Lessons learned from a volunteer program. *The Journal of Perinatal Education, 15*(3), 25–33. https://doi.org/10.1624/105812406X118995

Kayne, M. A., Greulich, M. B., & Albers, L. L. (2001). Doulas: an alternative yet complementary addition to care during childbirth. *Clinical obstetrics and gynecology, 44*(4), 692–703.

Kelaher, D., & Dollery, B. (2003). Health reform in China: an analysis of rural health care delivery. *Working Paper Series in Economics*. University of New England, School of Economic Studies. Retrieved from https://www.une.edu.au/__data/assets/pdf_file/0008/67859/econ-2003-17.pdf

Kennedy, H. P. (2000). A model of exemplary midwifery practice: Results of a Delphi study. *Journal of Midwifery & Women's Health, 45*(1), 4–19.

Kennedy, H. (2014). Foreword. In C. H. Morton & E. G. Clift (Eds.), *Birth Ambassadors: Doulas and the re-emergence of women-supported birth America* (pp. 21–23). Praeclarus Press.

Klaus, M. H., Kennell, J. H., & Klaus, P. H. (2002). *The doula book: How a trained labor companion can help you have a shorter, easier, and healthier birth*. Da Capo Press.

Kozhimannil, K. B., Johnson, P. J., Attanasio, L. B., Gjerdingen, D. K., & McGovern, P. M. (2013). Use of nonmedical methods of labor induction and pain management among U.S. women. *Birth, 40*(4), 227–236. https://doi.org/10.1111/birt.12064

Lamaze International Childbirth Education Instructor Training Handbook. (2017). Lamaze International Accredited Childbirth Program: The Pittsburgh Program.

Langer, A., Campero, L., Garcia, C., & Reynoso, S. (1998). Effects of psychosocial support during labour and childbirth on breastfeeding, medical interventions, and mothers' wellbeing in a Mexican public hospital: A randomised clinical trial. *British Journal of Obstetrics and Gynecology, 105*(10), 1056–1063.

Lazarus, E. S. (1994). What do women want?: Issues of choice, control, and class in pregnancy and childbirth. *Medical Anthropology Quarterly, 8*(1), 25–46.

Li, L., Chen, Q., & Powers, D. (2012). Chinese healthcare reform: A shift toward social development. *Modern China, 38*(6), 630–645. https://doi.org/10.1177/0097700412457913

Lindlof, T. R., & Taylor, B. C. (2011). *Qualitative communication research methods* (3rd ed.). Sage Publications.

Liu, Y. (2004). China's public health-care system: facing the challenges. *Bulletin of the World Health Organization, 82*(7), 532–538.

Liu, Y. P. (2005). *The beginning of the Chinese midwifery education and maternity care.* Retrieved from www.huliw.com/ad/lyp/33.Html

Liu, M. (2011). *Migration, prostitution, and human trafficking: The voice of Chinese women.* New Brunswick, New Jersey: Transaction Publishers.

Lothian, J. A. (2009). Safe, healthy birth: What every pregnant woman needs to know. *The Journal of Perinatal Education, 18*(3), 48–54.

Lupton, D. (1994). Toward the development of critical health communication praxis. *Health Communication, 6*(1), 55–67.

Ma, J., Lu, M., & Quan, H. (2008). From A national, centrally planned health system to A system based on the market: Lessons from china. *Health Affairs, 27*(4), 937–948. https://doi.org/10.1377/hlthaff.27.4.937

Ma, X. M., Chen, X. H., Wang, J. S., Lyman, G. H., Qu, Z., Ma, W., Song, J., Zhou, C., & Zhao, L. P. (2015). Evolving Healthcare Quality in Top Tertiary General Hospitals in China during the China Healthcare Reform (2010–2012) from the Perspective of Inpatient Mortality. *PloS one, 10*(12) Retrieved from http://journals.plos.org/plosone/article?id=10.1371/journal.pone.0140568

Martin, E. (2001). *The woman in the body: A cultural analysis of reproduction.* Beacon Press.

Milwertz, C. N. (1997). *Accepting population control: Urban Chinese women and the one-child family policy* (No. 74). Psychology Press.

Morgan, K. P. (1998). Contested Bodies, Contested Knowledges: Women, Health, and politics of Medicalization. In S. Sherwin (Ed.), *The politics of women's health: Exploring agency and autonomy* (pp. 83–121). Temple University Press.

Morse, J. M., & Field, P. A. (1995). *Nursing research: The application of qualitative approaches.* Nelson Thornes.

Morton, C. H., & Clift, E. (2014). *Birth Ambassadors: Doulas and the Re-emergence of Woman-Supported Birth America.* Praeclarus Press, LLC..

Neifert, M. R., & Seacat, J. M. (1986). Medical management of successful breast feeding. *Pediatric Clinics of North America, 33*(4), 743–762.

Papagni, K., & Buckner, E. (2006). Doula support and attitudes of intrapartum nurses: A qualitative study from the patient's perspective. *The Journal of Perinatal Education, 15*(1), 11–18. https://doi.org/10.1624/105812406X92949

Phillips, T. (2007). *Building the nation through women's health: Modern midwifery in early Twentieth-Century China* (Doctoral Dissertation). University of Pittsburg, PA. Retrieved from ProQuest.

Ramesh, M., Wu, X., & He, A. (2014). Health governance and healthcare reforms in China. *Health Policy and Planning, 29*(6), 663–672. https://doi.org/10.1093/heapol/czs109

Raven, J., van den Broek, N., Tao, F., Kun, H., & Tolhurst, R. (2015). The quality of childbirth care in China: women's voices: A qualitative study. *BMC Pregnancy and Childbirth, 15*(1), 113. Retrieved from https://bmcpregnancychildbirth.biomedcentral.com/articles/10.1186/s12884-015-0545-9

Sheffey, S. (2017). Women's Role in their Reproductive Process: The Effects of Authoritative Knowledge and Biomedical Interventions on the American Birth Experience. (Master Thesis). West Michigan University, MI. Retrieved from https://scholarworks.wmich.edu/masters_theses/913

Sherwin, S. (1998). *The politics of women's health: Exploring agency and autonomy.* Temple University Press.

Shu, Q., & Wang, D. (2002). Evaluation of Planning Childbirth. *Chinese Clinical Gynecology, 5,* 274–275. (in Chinese).

Sidel, V. W., & Sidel, R. (1974). *Serve the people: observations on medicine in the People's Republic of China.* Beacon Press.

Smith, R., & Tang, S. (2004). Nursing in China: Historical development, current issues and future challenges. *Japanese Journal of Nursing and Health Science, 5*(2), 16–20.

Srisuthisak, S. (2009). *Relationship among stress of labor, support, and childbirth experience in postpartum mothers* (Doctoral Dissertation). Virginia Commonwealth University, VA. Retrieved from ProQuest.

Stacey, J. (1997). *Teratologies: A cultural study of cancer.* Routledge.

Stange, M. Z., Oyster, C. K., & Sloan, J. E. (2011). *Encyclopedia of women in today's world.* Sage Publications.

Steel, A., Frawley, J., Adams, J., & Diezel, H. (2015). Trained or professional doulas in the support and care of pregnant and birthing women: a critical integrative review. *Health & Social Care in the Community, 23*(3), 225–241. https://doi.org/10.1111/hsc.12112

Stein, M. T., Kennell, J. H., & Fulcher, A. (2004). Benefits of a doula present at the birth of a child. *Journal of Developmental & Behavioral Pediatrics, 24,* 195–198.

Stevens, J., Dahlen, H., Peters, K., & Jackson, D. (2011). Midwives' and doulas' perspectives of the role of the doula in Australia: A qualitative study. *Midwifery, 27*(4), 509–516. https://doi.org/10.1016/j.midw.2010.04.002

Strauss, A., & Corbin, J. M. (1990). *Basics of qualitative research: Grounded theory procedures and techniques.* Sage Publications.

Sun, J., Wang, J., Wang, Z., Liu, Q., Liu, Y., Liu, S., . . . Ma, J. (2017). The impact of adverse media reporting on doctor–patient relationships in china: An analysis with propensity-score matching. *The Lancet, 390,* S100–S100. https://doi.org/10.1016/S0140-6736(17)33238-5

Tetteh, D. (2017). The breast cancer fanfare: Sociocultural factors and women's health in Ghana. *Health Care for Women International,* 1–18. https://doi.org/10.1080/07399332.2016.1215465

Tetteh, D. (2018). *Communication studies and feminist perspectives on ovarian cancer.* Lexington Books.

Treichler, P. A. (1990). Feminism, medicine, and the meaning of childbirth. In M. Jacobus, E. Keller, & S. Shuttleworth (Eds.), *Body/Politics: Women and the Discourses of Science* (pp.129–38). New York: Routledge.

Treichler, P. A. (2012). *How to have theory in an epidemic: Cultural chronicles of AIDS.* North Carolina: Duke University Press.

The Central Committee of the Chinese Communist Party (CPC) and the State Council on Further Strengthening Rural Health, "Decision". (October 19, 2002), Beijing, China.

Torres, J. (2013). Breast milk and labour support: Lactation consultants' and doulas' strategies for navigating the medical context of maternity care. *Sociology of Health & Illness, 35*(6), 924–938. https://doi.org/10.1111/1467-9566.12010

Tully, K. P., & Ball, H. L. (2014). Maternal accounts of their breast-feeding intent and early challenges after caesarean childbirth. *Midwifery, 30*(6), 712–719. https://doi.org/10.1016/j.midw.2013.10.014

Turshen, M. (2007). *Women's Health Movements: A Global force for change.* Springer Nature.

Wu, X., Liu, F. F., & Fang, P. Q. (2007). On the Reform in Corporate Governance Structure and Management System of Public Hospital. *Journal of Fujian Medical University (Social Science Edition), 2,* 1–5. (in Chinese).

Yu, L. (2014). *Chinese city and regional planning systems.* Ashgate Publishing Company.

Zauderer, C. (2009). Postpartum depression: How childbirth educators can help break the silence. *Journal of Perinatal Education, 18*(2), 23–31. https://doi.org/10.1624/105812409X426305

Zeng, Y., & Hesketh, T. (2016). The effects of China's universal two-child policy. *The Lancet, 388*(10054), 1930–1938. https://doi.org/10.1016/S0140-6736(16)31405-2

Zhai. Y. (2005). Doula – The friend and relative during the birth. *Healthy mother.* (In Chinese). Retrieved from http://baby.sina.com.cn/health/2005-03-03/47_69746.shtml

Zhang, Y. (2008). *Layered motherhood for Chinese mother bloggers: A feminist Foucauldian analysis* (Doctoral Dissertation). Bowling Green State University, OH. Retrieved from ProQuest.

Zheng, Y. (2010). Society must be defended: Reform, openness, and social policy in China. *Journal of Contemporary China, 19*(67), 799–818. https://doi.org/10.1080/10670564.2010.508579

Zheng, Y., Dong, S., & Lan, S. (2015). The Influence of Doula Instrument Combined with Doula Support to the Primiparas' Delivery. *Journal of International Obstetrics and Gynecology, 42*(5), 540–544. (in Chinese).

Zhou, L., Xu, X., Antwi, H., & Wang, L. (2017). Towards an equitable healthcare in China: Evaluating the productive efficiency of community health centers in Jiangsu province. *International Journal for Equity in Health, 16*. https://doi.org/10.1186/s12939-017-0586-y

Zhu, X., Lu, H., Hou, R., & Pang, R. (2015). Review of the midwifery related policies development progress in modern times of China. *Chinese Nursing Management, 15*(1), 122–125. (in Chinese).

Zraick, K. (2015, October 30). China will feel one-child policy's effects for decades, experts say. *The New York Times.* Retrieved from https://www.nytimes.com/2015/10/31/world/asia/china-will-feel-one-child-policys-effects-for-decades-experts-say.html

Chapter 2
Motivations for Chinese Women to Become Professional Doulas

For Chinese doulas in this study, the underlying motivation for becoming a doula was related directly to feeling called to support women in labor and being there with/for them. In fact, an "unhappy laboring experience" was a clear and strong motivation for Chinese doulas to get training and to become a professional doula. Chinese doulas that I interviewed pointed out that many maternity healthcare demands could not be fulfilled by the current Chinese maternal healthcare system. Likewise, one doula's working purpose was to "fill the gap" of the maternal healthcare system that failed women in labor.

Unhappy Labor Experiences

From the interviews I conducted and from the observation I had during my internship, I learned that women interested in becoming doulas and who did not work in the medical field or were not professional medical healthcare workers started to move toward doula care and childbirth education as their careers by learning perinatal knowledge during/after their pregnancies. One of the key themes that emerged from the interviews was the feeling that the current maternity system was failing women, and that many women had suffered through unhappy labor experiences. Unhappiness and painful labor experiences became a motivator for some Chinese women to study and embrace doula care in labor. They used phrases such as "bad experience" and "nightmare moment" to describe their childbirth experiences without doulas and doula care. Jian Ning, a mother doula, reflected on her labor experience with her first baby: "something was wrong with it" and "the night was a nightmare and [I] took [a] long time to recover from it." She was "very anxious" and wanted to have a doula with her, but she failed to find one. Jian Ning recalled her delivery experience as a "traumatized moment," and she said,

> My families had limited knowledge of childbirth, and they only held my hands to comfort me. My body was suffering the pain. I went to hospital in the early morning, and I did not go to the bathroom to pee until three or four in the afternoon. I did not know I could go to

This chapter is currently under the review and revision process for the *Journal of Women's Health International* the bathroom, and no one reminded me to do that. By the time one nurse informed me that I could go to the bathroom, there was something wrong with my bladder. Then the nurse connected the catheter for me. But it was too late. It was a nightmare for me that it took a long time for me to recover after the labor.

Similarly, Jiang Min, a mother doula, delivered her son about 4 years ago. When she recalled her delivery experience, she described it as a "desperate and hopeless moment." She said,

I had a very bad labor experience. I was about 41 weeks pregnant, but I did not have contractions by that time. My obstetrician injected the oxytocin into me, then I started to feel contraction pains. My obstetrician did nothing to me. She just let me lay on the bed. Then, I started to feel contractions, which was about three times every five minutes. I felt so desperate and hopeless at that moment...If there were a doula she would have been there with me; I would have felt much better instead of being isolated and lonely.

Meanwhile, Jiang Min said the "bad personal experience motivated me to start working as a doula" and that "I would like to bring support and company for women for their pregnancy and labor."

On the other hand, some women who have worked in medical institutions as midwives, nurses, or obstetricians started to embrace and apply doula care in their daily medical practices. Liu Ying graduated with a bachelor's degree in medicine. Afterward, she worked as an obstetrician in a public hospital for several years. She started to learn about the doula profession and doula care when she was pregnant in 2015. Liu Ying described her doula professional experience as "starting a new approach in obstetric study." Liu Ying stated,

I remembered there was a Wechat public account introduced in American obstetrician Barbara's (Barbara Harper) seminar in Beijing and her ideas of gentle birth. Then, I participated in her seminar as well as some related childbirth courses and doula trainings. I intended to apply the idea of doula care and gentle birth in my daily work. I introduced this idea to my colleagues and pregnant women since many of them did not realize the importance of this perspective.

Similarly, Wang Wei has worked as a licensed practical nurse in a government-based hospital since 2012. She delivered her baby in early 2016, but she "was terrified" during her laboring process and told me "it was painful." Wang Wei observed that one mom delivered a baby next to her using doula equipment.[1] She said,

At that time, I thought a doula was a medical instrument, which had two electronic connectors. The midwives and nurses told me the doula instrument could release the pain, but I did not know. I felt pain because of my contractions.

Having a medical background and being a new mother, Wang Wei learned about breastfeeding and then became a certified lactation consultant. She described both

---

[1] Chinese researchers have innovated a non-medical instrument for women to use in natural birth since 2000, and they named it "doula instrument" (*dao le yi qi* in Chinese). A news article published on *People's Daily* (2011) elaborated that a "doula instrument is an effective instrument for women to reduce pain labor. With the assistance of a doula instrument, the length of the labor is shortened to about 2 h in average." In this project, doula only refers to doula workers.

"being a mother and childbirth educator" as learning processes. Wang Wei also mentioned that her understanding of doulas began through medical training before she learned about doula care as a profession. She said,

> During the learning process, I knew that doula was not only an instrument but also a profession. The Lamaze Childbirth Educator Training seminar made me pay more attention to childbirth and respectful maternal healthcare. Reflecting on my personal labor experience, I would like to help other mothers in labor. I would like to provide doula support for them.

Wang Wei addressed the "painful and unhappy" experiences motivating her to continue her career as a licensed practical nurse as well as to improve women's labor experiences by helping them to "manage the release of the pains" as a doula and childbirth educator.

Filling the Gap: *I am with Her*

Currently, most labor suites in Chinese public hospitals (government-based) are always shared by other laboring mothers and are often considered too crowded and busy (Raven et al., 2015; Cheung et al., 2005). It is a fact that expectant mothers cannot receive adequate attention and support from the obstetrics staff in labor suites. Lin Jing, a mother doula, mentioned that she realized "there was something wrong" during her labor process, but all the obstetrics staff were too busy to listen and communicate with her. She said, "If I could have [had] a doula with me, there would have been a person to listen to me." Shen Yu, a hospital-based doula, talked about her understanding of the current Chinese hospital-based labor suite, and she said,

> It is the fact that we are always in shortage of hands in the labor suite. On one hand, we have many doctors and nurses, but only a few of them choose to work in the obstetrics department. One delivery room only has three or four midwives, but it will have about 20 expectant women in labor. It is impossible to ask midwives and obstetricians to provide continuous support for every single expectant woman in labor. On the other hand, doulas can help midwives and obstetricians' work by providing doula care for expectant mothers. Doulas can spend adequate time to talk with expectant mothers, and it is verbal encouragement. Doulas also can provide physical support. For instance, I always do massages for women to help release the pain.

From the perspective of most of the Chinese doulas I interviewed, the role of doulas is supposed to "fill the gap by talking with the mothers and providing massages when the expectant mothers needed it."

Moreover, many doulas believed that when they came to the labor suites to attend to the mothers the mothers would not feel alone or be isolated. He Pei, an obstetrician, lactation consultant, and doula, shared her thoughts on helping women through the feeling of isolation. She said,

> Many pregnant women mentioned they were afraid of the pains in labor. Besides the fear of pains, I think many of them feel uncomfortable in the labor suite because it is a strange location. It is a natural reaction. Doulas (in the delivery room) could reduce women's

feeling of isolation and the uncertainties in the labor process. It is a common sense that having a person you trust by your side would be great in the unfamiliar place.

In fact, the companionship that the doulas provided extended beyond the delivery suite. Through social media and related communication technologies, doulas report that they are always accessible (through WeChat, telephone phone, or face-to-face communication) to support women for as long as they needed, even for future pregnancies. Huang Ru, a doula and childbirth educator, worked with a 33-week pregnant mother. She said,

> From the moment she (the mother) confirmed having me as her doula until she delivered the baby, we talked a lot. In our daily face-to-face communication and Wechat/telephone talk, she thought my words were very powerful. I believe that I should be with them—the mothers, whenever they need me.

Similarly, Wang Wei established a WeChat group for expectant mothers and women who planned to have babies in the future. She said that there were more than 250 women in her group, and she encouraged them to share experiences and to raise concern and questions relating to maternity (e.g., pregnancy and breastfeeding) in the group. In Wang Wei's opinion, "The online communication group could be a good communication platform for mothers. They can learn from me as well as from each other." Additionally, Shen Yu mentioned that she always tried to meet and communicate with expectant mothers at least 3 months before the due dates. Just as Shen Yu said, "They could contact me anytime. I am with them all the time, so I think we are families and friends."

On one hand, the Chinese women's motivations for becoming doulas were broadly consistent with Lantz's research (2005) and Hardeman and Kozhimannil's study (2016), which focused on American doulas and pregnant women. Hardeman and Kozhimannil found that most women wanted to become doulas in order to support and empower other women. Through the interviews, I gained a unique understanding of the Chinese doula workforce and doulas' support for Chinese women during pregnancy and labor.

Many interviewees associated "fear of pain in labor," "feeling of being left out," "isolation," "disappointment and hopelessness," "no company in the labor suite," and "no emotional support" with "bad labor experiences." Jian Ning, one of the participants in this study, mentioned that she realized that "there was something wrong" in the pre-delivery room, but all the obstetrics staff were too busy to listen and communicate with her. Jian Ning did not know she could go to the bathroom to urinate. Jian Ning said,

> No one told me I could go to the bathroom, and I did not know. I tried to ask them [obstetrics staff], but no one talked to me. I did not urinate for more than 6–7 hours. When a nurse reminded me that I could urinate in labor, my body did not function anymore.

As a result, Jian Ning got a urinary tract infection (UTI). Like Jian Ning, both Jiang Min and Wang Wei also described their labors as "bad experiences" and "traumatized memories." In fact, the "bad labor experiences" were partially caused by inadequate attention and maternal care from midwives, nurses, and obstetricians in the delivery rooms.

What I have observed in WeCare WMH is that in the private maternal hospitals expectant mothers could choose to labor in a single labor suite and then receive adequate attention in labor. At WeCare WMH, for instance, for one birth mother there are about nine obstetrics staff members working with her, including two obstetricians, two midwives, two nurses, two pediatricians, and one doula[2] (Field observation, May ninth, 2017). However, almost all labor suites in Chinese public hospitals (government-based) are shared by other laboring mothers and are often considered too crowded and busy (Raven et al., 2015; Cheung et al., 2005). Laboring mothers cannot receive adequate attention and support from obstetrics staff. Therefore, I suggest that Chinese doulas could support obstetrics staff in the delivery rooms (especially government-based public hospitals) by filling obstetrics staff labor shortages in labor suites. Chinese doulas could also facilitate mothers' coping with childbirth in ways that the current Chinese maternal healthcare system (and midwives, obstetricians, and nurses) are unable to offer.

Interestingly, these "bad labor experiences" also became an opportunity to motivate Chinese women to learn about pregnancy and childbirth, regardless of whether they had a medical education background or not. Lin Jing said she started to read related books and articles about childbirth and labor. She stated,

> There were many questions and problems that could not be answered by others. The obstetricians lacked patience after I asked hundreds of questions, and they did not exactly know about my feelings. All these motivated me to study in obstetrics, although I did not receive any education in medical school. Of course,   what I have learned is very little and I absolutely need to catch up more.

Like Lin Jing, women interested in childbirth who dedicated themselves to the doula care profession also read a lot of medical textbooks, which were normally taught by Chinese medical schools. In the interviews, Xue Li, a mother doula, mentioned she had studied pathology for several months and was preparing to take a test. Both Lin Jing and Xue Li read books according to their interests and needs during their doula care work. As Xue Li said, "There will be some situations that I have not encountered before, and I am aware that I lack knowledge in some cases. Thus, I want to study as much as possible."

Chinese doulas who did not receive institutional higher education training in medical or related fields, but who have the strong desire for being good mothers and doulas in order to help other women have good labor experiences, were also driven to study in childbirth, labor, and related obstetrics areas. Lin Jing also mentioned that she viewed expectant mothers as her sisters, and sometimes she even viewed them as herself. This kind of strong psychological reflection also motivated many Chinese women to choose doula care as their profession. Meanwhile, doulas like Liu Ying and Wang Wei received degrees in medicine-related areas and have worked in clinics or hospitals, so they viewed doula-attended childbirth as an effective approach to avoid a "bad labor experience" and an opportunity to address women's biological and emotional needs in labor.

---

[2] The costs differ tremendously between laboring at a public and a private hospital.

Morton and Clift (2014) suggested that pregnant women expect to receive support from obstetrics staff. However, obstetrics staff often fail to provide adequate emotional, informational, or physical support to pregnant women in labor (Tumblin & Simkin, 2001). Even worse, American nurses spent less than 10% of their time providing emotional support for pregnant women in labor (Morton & Clift, 2014; Korst, Eusebio-Angeja, Chamorro, Aydin, & Gregory, 2003).

From my field research and interviews, I gained a general sense that, similar to American obstetrics sittings, Chinese pregnant women in labor rarely receive emotional support from obstetricians, midwives, or nurses. Pregnant women were sometimes left out in delivery rooms (Field observation, May 20th, 2017). Some doulas also expressed an inclination to choose the doula care profession as "intentions to fill the gap with continuous support when the expectant mothers needed it" in labor. Guided by the international doulas' associations, Chinese doulas provide expectant mothers in labor with emotional support (e.g., comforting and encouraging words, such as "believe yourself," "listen to your body," "you will be great"), informational support (e.g., informing expectant mothers about different labor stages, providing information of induction and usage of epidural once suggested by obstetricians), and physical support (e.g., provision of massages for expectant mothers' legs and backs, helping them walk around the delivery room based on expectant mothers' willingness). In addition, Chinese doulas also believed their presence in labor suites would decrease the mothers' feelings of fear and isolation, which provides a significant portion of emotional support. Like Jian Ning said,

> The labor suite is an unfamiliar place for an expectant mother. She could be anxious and uncomfortable by herself. When I am with her, she will be calmed because we have a trustworthy relationship and emotional connection. I think physically being with them means quite a lot.

Moreover, the companionship that Chinese doulas provide goes beyond the boundaries of the delivery suites. As Shen Yu and Wang Wei mentioned, they were always reachable through various communication channels for women during pregnancy, the approaching due date, and the postpartum period. On one hand, the doulas' high reachability distinguished them from hospital-based midwives and obstetricians who rarely gave their personal contact information to pregnant women. In the interviews, I found that high reachability was also generated by WeChat—a massive Chinese social media network and an instant messaging app. By March 2018, WeChat had reached 1 billion users globally (Ong, 2018). The prevalence of WeChat among Chinese people in their daily lives contributed to the doulas' 24/7 availability to pregnant women. Also, with WeChat, doulas have capabilities to connect all the pregnant women they know to a virtual group. Within online groups, pregnant women are able to ask questions about pregnancy and labor, and doulas can provide professional consultations for expectant mothers through texts, audio messages, or video calls. By using WeChat and other related interactive communication technologies (e.g., Weibo, QQ), doulas fill support gaps by providing the kinds of support (e.g., informational support, emotional support) that obstetrics staff in hospitals cannot offer to pregnant women.

On the other hand, many Chinese doulas also worked as lactation consultants who provided breastfeeding advice for women in the postpartum period. In other words, they served as birth doulas for pregnant women, and then they worked as lactation consultants for these new mothers during postnatal care. For instance, Wang Wei, Jiang Min, Jain Ning, Xue Meimei, and Zeng Rui described themselves as lactation consultants. For some of the interviewees, they explained that their paths to careers in childbirth education began with working as lactation consultants.

Generally, lactation consultants provided individual, face-to-face and professional counseling on breastfeeding (Clifford & McIntyre, 2008; Binns et al., 2003). One of the participants, Shen Yu, informed me that many Chinese lactation consultants initially started to work as *cuirushi*. *Cuirushi* is a person who assists a mother to produce more breast milk volume by massaging their breasts. However, Chinese Ministry of Human Resources do not recognize *cuirushi* as a category of job (Ouyang et al., 2016), and registering with government authorities as *cuirushi* was not required. Shen Yu said, "Many women start to work as *cuirushi* at the beginning of their career in maternal healthcare since it is easy to master the massaging and therapy skills." However, since Chinese authorities have started to discipline the industry of maternal health workers, many *cuirushi* have started to participate in relevant professional training about breastfeeding in order to receive certifications in lactation and breastfeeding consulting. A large number of the study participants were certified lactation consultants. Xue Li told me that she was certified as an International Board of Lactation Consultant (hereafter IBCLC). "I took breastfeeding seminars at Beijing on behalf of the IBCLC. After that, I passed the exam and became a certified lactation consultant," Xue Li said.

Based on the interviews, it is possible to see that Chinese doulas play multiple roles as maternal healthcare workers. The support they provide is continuous and consistent, which extends beyond the time of pregnancy and labor into the postpartum period. Both Shen Yu and He Pei mentioned that they would stay in touch with the mothers they had worked with. "If these mothers would plan to have another child(ren), I would like to be their doula again," Shen Yu said.

It is worth to note one of the most important reasons for Chinese women to enter the doula care profession was their personal labor experience. The "nightmare labor experience" motivated many women to work as doulas to support other women in labor. Chinese doulas pointed out that one of their working goals was to "fill the gap" of the maternal healthcare system that failed women in labor. Chinese doulas were able to provide different types of support (e.g., emotional, information, and physical support) in the labor suites in order to fill the care gaps that obstetricians and midwives could not fulfill. Importantly, what made Chinese doulas unique as maternal healthcare workers was their prevalent utilization of communication technologies, particularly WeChat, which enabled them to establish continuous supportive communication among pregnant women and experienced mothers. Likewise, the care Chinese doulas provide extends past the boundaries of time (pregnancy and labor) and physical locations (labor suites).

References

Binns, C. W., Li, L., & Zhang, M. (2003). Chinese mothers' knowledge and attitudes about breast-feeding in Perth, Western Australia. *Breastfeeding Review, 11*(3), 13.

Cheung, N. F., Mander, R., & Cheng, L. (2005). The 'doula-midwives' in Shanghai. *Evidence Based Midwifery, 3*(2), 73–80.

Clifford, J., & McIntyre, E. (2008). Who supports breastfeeding? *Breastfeeding Review, 16*(2), 9–19.

Hardeman, R. R., & Kozhimannil, K. B. (2016). Motivations for entering the doula profession: Perspectives from women of color. *Journal of Midwifery & Women's Health, 61*, 773–780. https://doi.org/10.1111/jmwh.12497

Korst, L., Eusebio-Angeja, A., Chamorro, T., Aydin, C., & Gregory, K. (2003). Nursing documentation time during implementation of an electronic medical record. *Journal of Nursing Administration, 33*(1), 24–30.

Lantz, P. M., Low, L. K., Varkey, S., & Watson, R. L. (2005). Doulas as childbirth paraprofessionals: Results from a national survey. *Women's Health Issues, 15*(3), 109–116. https://doi.org/10.1016/j.whi.2005.01.002

Morton, C. H., & Clift, E. (2014). *Birth ambassadors: Doulas and the re-emergence of woman-supported birth America*. Praeclarus Press, LLC.

Ong, T. (2018, March 5). *Chinese social media platform Wechat reaches 1 billion accounts worldwide*. The Verge. Retrieved from https://www.theverge.com/2018/3/5/17080546/wechat-chinese-social-media-billionusers-china

Ouyang, Y., Su, M., & Redding, S. R. (2016). A survey on difficulties and desires of breast feeding women in Wuhan, China. *Midwifery, 37*, 19–24. https://doi.org/10.1016/j.midw.2016.03.014

Raven, J., van den Broek, N., Tao, F., Kun, H., & Tolhurst, R. (2015). The quality of childbirth care in China: women's voices: A qualitative study. *BMC Pregnancy and Childbirth, 15*(1), 113. Retrieved from https://bmcpregnancychildbirth.biomedcentral.com/articles/10.1186/s12884-015-0545-9

Tumblin, A., & Simkin, P. (2001). Pregnant women's perceptions of their nurse's role during labor and delivery. *Birth, 28*(1), 52–56.

Chapter 3
Sisterhood: Sisters and Friends

With the work of Robin Morgan's *Sisterhood Is Powerful: An Anthology of Writings from the Women's Liberation Movement* (1971), the second-wave feminist movement appealed to "sisterhood to forge widespread solidarity among all women" (Qi, 2010, p. 328; Li, 2010). Sisterhood is defined as the "solidarity of women based on shared conditions, experiences, or concerns" (Hooks, 1986; Simmonds, 1997). Since then, the idea of sisterhood has moved beyond a biological definition to encapsulate social support between women across differences (Dill, 1983; Carby, 2007). Sisterhood relationships, therefore, could be described as a close friendship or bond between women (Qi, 2010; Husband, 2015; Carby, 2007). The development of sisterhood or close friendships bonds signifies the strong ties that exist among women.

Further, the health and wellness benefits of female friendship have been wide-ranging topics as the relationships among women can serve as catalysts for the improvement of women's health conditions (see Husband, 2015; Tatum, 2017; Branca, 2013). A large number of studies suggest that sisterhood among women is more likely to improve women's health, reduce stress, and create happiness (see Netuveli et al., 2006; Umberson & Montez, 2010; Ramos, 2012). Within these friendships, friends have relatively equal influence over each other, listen to each other's demands, foster good health, and provide the support and emotional confirmation that friends need (Blieszner, 2014; Samter, 2003; Verderber & MacGeorge, 2016).

Social support is defined as the assistance that we provide to others who we believe need our aid (Verderber & MacGeorge, 2016). Adding to that, Shumaker and Brownell (1984) define social support as "an exchange of resources between at least two individuals perceived by the provider or the recipient to be intended to enhance the wellbeing of the recipient" (p. 13). A growing body of research has indicated that social support is linked with important health outcomes, including better recovery from illness, longer life, reduced risk of disease, and an improved ability to cope with chronic illness and a variety of stressors (Burleson & MacGeorge,

Z. Z. Dai, *Maternal Healthcare and Doulas in China*,
https://doi.org/10.1007/978-3-030-46963-4_3

2002; MacGeorge et al., 2011; Stana & Flynn, 2012; Hanasono & Yang, 2016). For instance, emotional support (e.g., companionship, attentive listening, sympathy, expression of affection) can help to relieve emotional distress, and informational support (e.g., information and advice) can help recipients engage in educated problem-solving (see Greif & Sharpe, 2010; Brennan & Fink, 2013; Dubois & Loisell, 2009).

As I discussed in Chap. 2, Chinese pregnant women sometimes were left out in labor suites because labor suites were crowded and busy with several pregnant women but fewer obstetricians and midwives. Pregnant women do not receive adequate emotional attention and support from obstetrics staff (e.g., obstetricians, midwives, nurses). Furthermore, I find that many Chinese doulas are able to provide continuous support for pregnant women in labor (see details in Chap. 3). In fact, the provision of social support by Chinese doulas is not limited to emotional support, but also has extended to informational support, physical support, advice, and more. Because Chinese doulas' social support is intended to "fill the gap that [the] current maternal hospital system cannot provide," it is important to understand the provision of social support from a relational perspective, specifically in terms of sisterhood and female friendships.

Essentially, social support in the form of a sisterhood relationship can provide a buffer against stressful conditions and negative major life transitions that women experience in life (Husband, 2015; Pascoe & Richman, 2009; Jones & Wirtz, 2006). As I noted in the previous chapters, pregnancy and childbirth are unique times for women in general, and women may experience emotional changes and physically suffer from pain and discomfort (Morton, & Clift, 2014). Therefore, women need to receive support from close friends, family, and intimate partners (normally, their husbands) during pregnancy and childbirth.

McCubbin and Patterson (1983) suggest that the presence and support of families and close friends is conducive to a person's well-being, overall health, and ability to cope with challenging situations (Institution of Medicine, 2018; Remmers et al., 2010). As I note in previous chapters, for various reasons the husbands and close families of pregnant Chinese women were not allowed to enter labor suites to provide support in childbirth. To some extent, Chinese doulas play the significant role of "being the company" for women in labor.

In fact, Chinese doulas in this study talked about their close relationships with expectant mothers using such terms and phrases as "sisters," "close friends," and "like family." Because these terms and phrases emerged thematically in the interviews, I analyze the discourse of sisterhood and close relationships in this chapter. In addition, I note that a sense of sisterhood is central for many Chinese doulas and expectant mothers and show how some doulas view their work as the provision of social support to expectant mothers.

Sisterhood Is Strong and Powerful: Sisters, Friends, and Love

Unlike traditional paid or unpaid employment relationships between healthcare workers and patients, Chinese doulas characterized their relationships with expectant mothers as "families," "close friends," and "sisters." He Pei, an obstetrician and doula, explained the relationships between herself and the mothers she has worked with as similar to "a good and very close family" because they trusted each other. He Pei said,

> This type of close relationship is very easy to understand. I support and am there with them in the most difficult and challenging moment in their lives. It is certain that we will be close friends and families. It is a natural interaction.

Meanwhile, Jian Ning, a mother doula, noted that the pregnant women she has worked with are like her younger sisters to her. Jian Ning said,

> Sometimes I treat an expectant mother as my younger sister, and sometimes I think she is another "me." Sometimes, I tear up when I see the baby. I am happy for the mother and her baby.

Similarly, Lin Jing, a mother doula, also described her experiences with the mothers she worked with in terms of sisterhood. She stated,

> Those mothers I have worked with are my sisters. I could not say they will remember me for the rest of their lives, but they definitely could remember me for a long time. It is like an old Chinese saying about offering fuel in snowy weather—timely support, and I am happy to be with them too.

Importantly, many Chinese doulas also emphasized trust and respect in their sisterhood relationships with expectant mothers. He Pei stated, "The most significant thing between doulas and mothers is about trust. Once a mother fully trusts me (a doula), she could follow my lead in childbirth." She also believed that trustfulness increased the closeness in a doula's relationship with an expectant mother. Likewise, Ming Jing, a registered experienced nurse and doula, articulated the relationships between doulas and expectant mothers as "interdependent trust." She said,

> Doulas have to understand expectant mothers from both psychological and physiological perspectives since women in labor are very sensitive.

Ming Jing mentioned that within "interdependent trust relationships" expectant women in labor were more likely to have a satisfactory experience.

Jiang Min, a mother doula, described her perception of sisterhood relationships with expectant mothers as "love." She said,

> Once you choose this profession, you must embrace love in your work. Otherwise, you probably will leave this job after a few years. If a woman only wants to make money and she works as a doula, she will not persist in working in it. The reason that many women dedicate their careers to the doula profession is due to love and their willingness to help other women in childbirth.

Jiang Min also described her doula work with expectant mothers as a chance and as "*yuanfen*," which can be understood philosophically as karma. She stated,

It was a beautiful chance for me to meet them and their babies. I valued this kind of karma a lot. Despite how they evaluated my support in labor, I worked as best I could. They were my sisters.

Huang Ru, another mother doula, described her understanding of the relationship between doulas and mothers as "a love sisterhood relationship." She equated the doula profession with a "great love." "Doula is a profession of great love. Without love, you could not be a qualified doula."

Many Chinese doulas noted that they believed that childbirth is "a turning point for women in their lives since it was an opportunity for them to start to recognize their capabilities" as well as "a good opportunity for expectant mothers to think about their lives." Xue Li, a doula and lactation consultant, shared her doula profession working stories. She said,

Many mothers shared their birth stories with me. One message these women shared was that they felt different when they insisted on having a natural delivery. They believed that they made the decisions themselves and listened to their bodies. I knew a large number of women were not very clear about their lives in terms of careers or families. They always listened to other persons, including their parents, husbands, or in-laws. In my opinion, childbirth became a wakeful moment for many women. They started to believe themselves and became more confident as well as strong. According to my personal experiences, a few women started to reflect on their lives when they got divorced, which was very sad. Making decisions on natural birth empowered women, and they believed that they were not subjects anymore. Also, women started to realize their capabilities. I just think that is amazing.

Also, Lin Jing believed that a doula served as "a coach and psychological consultant" for pregnant women, who helped pregnant women to take responsibility for themselves and informed them about empowerment. Lin Jing stated,

Some expectant mothers asked me whether they should have an epidural or not; and some of them asked me whether they should insist on natural birth or not, especially when they had a C-section for their first babies or their obstetricians suggested they choose C-section. When they asked me questions, I told them to listen to their bodies and make the decisions themselves. I told them "do not listen to me, and do not listen to your families." I think they should start to learn to be themselves and take responsibility for themselves. Childbirth is a turning point for many of them.

Chinese doulas in this study spoke of their relationships with expectant mothers as sisters, families, and close friends. Different from the typical professional relationships between healthcare givers and their clients or patients, Chinese doulas form intimate relationships with expectant mothers. "They are my sisters and families" and "we are good friends" were repeatedly stated by many Chinese doulas. Their perception of being "families," "sisters," and "friends" reflects the idea that "modern social arrangements have redefined the importance of friendship and the functions it served" (Allan, 2008; Castaneda & Burns-Glover, 2008). In other words, the concept of "family" has expanded and is reflected within the discourse of sisterhood relationships between Chinese doulas and expectant mothers. The statement "we are sisters" also refers to sibling relationships, which normally can span a longer time than other family relationships (Myers & Kennedy-Lightsey, 2015; Verderber & MacGeorge, 2016). Therefore, we see that Chinese women have created families and sisterly bonds through various emotional and supportive ties. In terms of Chinese doulas and their provision of doula care to expectant mothers, we see that the professional caregiving relationships between them have transformed into family relationships with certain caring functions and services.

Women's friendships incorporate many shared activities, which involve self-disclosure and emotional support for each other (Verderber & MacGeorge, 2016). Peirce (1958) points out that we cannot separate our ideas from our experiences, knowers from knowledge, for there is an inseparable connection between rational cognition and rational purpose, between thoughts and action, between thinking and doing (Qi, 2010). Therefore, sisterhood relationships between doulas and expectant mothers highlight how shared childbirth experiences connect women as a unified group. Concerning many Chinese women's motivations for working as doulas (see the previous chapter), the common experiences of childbirth and beginning the journey of motherhood have led Chinese doulas and expectant mothers to stand in solidarity.

Moreover, the doulas' and expectant mothers' sisterhood relationships represent trust and respect, which could facilitate pregnant women's feelings of safety and certainty working with Chinese doulas (Caiazza & Putnam, 2005; Putnam, 2001; Son et al., 2010; Blackshaw & Long, 2005). Regarding their own mothers' identities, Chinese doulas always felt for other pregnant women. Like Jian Ning said, "Sometimes, I think she is another 'me' who is going to deliver the baby." In fact, Jian Ning is putting herself into someone else's position and experiencing what she is feeling, which can be described as one type of empathy—perspective taking (Toto et al., 2015). Following my interviews, I understand that many Chinese doulas present an ability to emotionally "resonate" with other's feeling by empathizing her own child birthing experience. The emotional resonance between doulas and birthing mothers originates from doulas' personal laboring experiences and their motivations to practice doula care. On one hand, they are similar to "old-wives" or "birth nannies" midwifery who provide maternity healthcare to birthing mothers in indigenous times; they also do not have institutional medicalization training and provide labor support based on their individual childbirth experiences. On the other hand, Chinese doulas are different from "old-wives" midwifery because their companionship and guidance for birthing mothers are regulated. Importantly, doulas are not making decisions for birthing women like the "old-wives" used to do. Doulas are not in charge of the childbirth process; instead, they focus on facilitating emotional and informational support for women in labor. The goal of doula care is to empower women's bodies and agencies in labor. Therefore, the emotions of trust, respect, and empathy create special opportunities for intimate communication between Chinese doulas and birthing mothers.

It is worth pointing out that many Chinese doulas mentioned that a pregnant woman's socioeconomic status had a big impact on their communication. In terms of pregnant women who came from less developed regions or who did not receive higher education, doulas had to "spend more time to communicate with them and explain things in detail." Qin Nan also explained that "doulas needed to elaborate things clearly" instead of "just informing the idea of healthy birth" since this group of women took more time to accept new concepts. Just as she said,

> For instance, one of the mothers I worked with mentioned she was under the pain of contractions, and she asked me whether she should keep lying there or stand up or have some liberal positions. We had talked about liberal positions all the time. I thought she could listen to her body and move herself. However, she still had some concerns. For this situation, I (as a doula) needed to practice good interpersonal communication by talking with her.

Although many Chinese doulas had socioeconomic and educational differences in relation to the expectant mothers they worked with, many Chinese doulas in this study were able to overcome barriers associated with these differences by perceiving other women's thoughts and feelings of pregnancy and childbirth. In my opinion, the symbolic ideas of sisterhood and friendships among Chinese doulas and expectant mothers came up in the shared experiences of pregnancy and labor, which became the "main components of sorority memberships among women" (Whaley, 2010, p.122).

Concerning Chinese women's motivations to work as doulas, I found that the women I interviewed each had a strong desire to enhance women's empowerment in the context of childbirth as well as more broadly in their lives. Friendships and sisterhood between women could be empowering when close connections and ties are constructed with someone who is trusted, when there is a clear understanding of plights, struggles, and triumphs, and when relational bonds are linked with physical and psychological health conditions (Blieszner, 2014; Cable et al., 2013; Husband, 2015). In this study, pregnancy and the experience of childbirth could be viewed as "struggles and triumphs" for Chinese women, including both doulas and expectant mothers. Like Wang Wei said, "It is a triumph when both mother and her baby are safe." Chinese doulas' recognition of the importance of childbirth was an attentive moment for Chinese women in general since they started to "listen to their bodies, trust their determinations, and made decisions for themselves" instead of just obeying or depending on their husbands or families.

What Have We Missed—Sister, Family or Emotional Labour[1]?

As I introduced in the previous section, Ming Jing—a former experienced nurse and current doula—described the relationships between doulas and birthing mothers as "interdependent trust." She viewed the birthing mothers as her sisters, good friends, and family members. In the interview, Ming Jing also informed me that many pregnant women and their families called her "Aunt Ming" (*Ming yi* in Chinese). Ming Jing said,

---

[1] Guided by Arlie Hochschild's work, I use the term "labour" instead of "labor" in this section since I provide a discussion regarding the theory of "emotional labour." Moreover, the book follows U.S. spellings of "labour", and I do not change labour to labor in the section for the word 'emotional labour'.

Some people might not know my full name. However, when you mention "Aunt Ming," everyone knows that is me. "Aunt Ming" is one of the most popular obstetrics staff in this hospital. I have been told that many birthing mothers in labor suites wanted to see me, although I was not on duty at that time. Some birthing mothers directly tell their obstetricians or midwives that they would like to see "Aunt Ming" before laboring. They really trust me, and I know I am able to comfort them. To be honest, I would like to help them to release fears before labor. When I work as a doula, I am happy. I love to bring happiness to birthing mothers, and I love to be an aunt for all women (in this hospital). I am grateful to be a doula when I see a woman deliver a baby safely. Sometimes, a woman and her family would give me some candies after her labor. They celebrate their family event with me. However, I am also nervous. Every day, I hear birthing women complain about pains in labor, I see their tears, and I know their fears. I am anxious, too. I am afraid I am not able to provide good doula care service for them. I do not want to disappoint them.

Ming Jing enjoyed working with birthing mothers, but she also struggled emotionally. She mentioned that she never expressed any negative emotions at work, although she did have some bad days. Ming Jing said,

I remembered that one morning (months ago) my car was hit by another car on the way to work, and I was mad. However, I did not say anything at work. I maintained a smiling face when I saw the mothers. When a woman comes to the hospital to deliver her baby, it is a life-changing event for her and her families. They are happy, and I want to be happy for/ with them.

I shared Ming Jing's concerns and anxieties. From the interviews I conducted and my observation at WeCare WMH, I have learned that pregnancy and child birthing are emotionally charged experiences (also see Hunter, 2001). Arlie Hochschild (1979, 1983) defines emotion work as the effort people invest in managing their own emotions and the way that individuals manage their feelings. Hochschild also acknowledges that what people feel and what is communicated is influenced by socially constructed "feeling rules" (Hochschild, 1979, p. 563; 1983, 2000). "Feeling rules" direct how people "want to try to feel" (Hochschild, 1979, p. 563). In any given situation, people engage in "surface" or "deep" acting to manage their emotions by presenting "what [people] expect to feel with idealization" (Hochschild, 1979, p. 565). Hochschild also notes that "'emotion work' refers to the effort—the act of trying—and not to the outcome" (p. 561). She suggests that when emotions are managed, when "on stage performing" or "deep acting," most individuals are not aware of how much emotion work they invest (p. 561).

I could not help thinking of Ming Jing regarding how much emotion work she invests in her doula care work. I did not know if it was easy for her to manage her feelings (mad and angry) when her car was hit because she still *smiled* to everyone and acted *happy* at work. I did not know when Ming Jing saw birthing mothers' tears and listened to their fears regarding labor—yet, did anyone think about *her*? When a birthing mother is excited to share her happiness of having a son or daughter with Aunt Ming, does anyone ask her "how are you doing?" or "have you had a good day?" Perhaps birthing mothers and families are just eager to share all of their emotions with Aunt Ming because she is always *happy, smiling, lovely, respectful, supportive,* and *she is a family member.* Alternatively, Ming Jing may be just like the midwives in John and Parsons' (2006) study who is "putting on a professional face" for most of the time (p. 268).

Midwives, maternity healthcare workers, and doulas revealed their emotional burnout in supporting women in labor (see Naiman-Sessions et al., 2017; Carlise et al., 1994; John & Parsons, 2006). In John and Parsons' (2006) article, *Shadow Work in Midwifery: Unseen and Unrecognized Emotional Labour*, they find that

> The midwives reported that the emotional labour involved was draining and stressful, but they felt it was necessary to provide the emotional care needed by women. For mothers, maintaining normality during birth was important, with little recognition of the e m o - tional work involved, for them it was seen as a prerequisite of the job…. (p. 266)

Hochschild (1983) defines the concept of emotional labour as "the management of feeling to create publicly observable facial and bodily display" (p.7). The theory of emotional labour is underpinned by Marxist theory, which challenges the commodification of feelings in an organizational setting and the way workers' feelings can be manipulated or exploited for financial reasons (Hochschild, 1983). In Arlie Hochschild's article, *Global Care Chains and Emotional Surplus Value*, Hochschild writes (2000),

> Global capitalism affects whatever it touches, and it touches virtually everything including what I call global care chains—a series of personal links between people across the globe based on the paid or unpaid work. Usually, women make up these chains. (p.131)

Therefore, emotional labour theory is also underpinned by feminist theory, which critiques the general expectations that emotion work is women's work (Hochschild, 2000, 2003). "Caring work touches people's emotions. It is emotional labour, and [it is] partly visible, partly invisible" (Hochschild, 2000, p.134). James (1989, 1992) further emphasizes that working in a healthcare environment, the effort of managing feelings or emotions is invisible and unacknowledged.

A doula is in a special position in relation to women's child birthing procedures. As I examined in the previous chapters, doulas are a unique group of maternity healthcare workers different from obstetricians, midwives, and nurses. Many women work as doulas because they have a motivation to care for other women in laboring and have a belief in love and caring. Like Ming Jing, many of them might be very good at managing their emotions with various coping strategies. Many doulas might also be called "Aunt Ming" or "Mother Ming," and they always try to maintain normality and establish a loving and happy environment for birthing mothers since a calm environment has positive effects on women's labor (Hodnett et al., 2007). However, what have we missed?

What we have missed is Ming Jing always replies to an expectant mother's WeChat or text message in five minutes, and her quick response is taken for granted.

What we have missed is Ming Jing's tears when she had a bad day.

What we have missed is Ming Jing's anxieties and fears.

What we have missed is a doula working non-stop for more than 20 hours to provide support for another woman.

What we have missed is a doula may feel emotionally burned out.

What we have missed is a doula's large amount of unseen work regarding emotion management and professional performance. What we have missed is only defining a doula and a birthing mother as sisters but never question the intimate relationship.

References

Allan, G. (2008). Flexibility, friendship, and family. *Personal Relationships, 15*(1), 1–16.
Blackshaw, T., & Long, J. (2005). What's the big idea? A critical exploration of the concept of social capital and its incorporation into leisure policy discourse. *Leisure Studies, 24*(3), 239–258.
Blieszner, R. (2014). The worth of friendship: Can friends keep us happy and healthy? *Generations-Journal of the American Society on Aging, 38*(1), 24–30.
Branca, P. (2013). *Silent sisterhood: Middle-class women in the Victorian home*. Routledge.
Brennan, P. F., & Fink, S. V. (2013). Health promotion, social support, and computer networks. In R. L. Street, W. R. Gold, & T. Manning (Eds.), *Health promotion and interactive technology: Theoretical applications and future directions* (pp. 157–170). Routledge.
Burleson, B. R., & MacGeorge, E. L. (2002). Supportive communication. *Handbook of interpersonal communication, 3*, 374–424.
Cable, N., Bartley, M., Chandola, T., & Sacker, A. (2013). Friends are equally important to men and women, but family matters more for men's well-being. *Journal of Epidemiology and Community Health, 67*(2), 166–171. https://doi.org/10.1136/jech-2012-201113
Caiazza, A., & Putnam, R. D. (2005). Women's status and social capital in the United States. *Journal of Women, Politics & Policy, 27*(1-2), 69–84. https://doi.org/10.1300/J501v27n01_05
Carby, H. (2007). White woman listen! Black feminism and the boundaries of sisterhood. In A. Gray, J. Campbell, M. Erickson, S. Hanson, & H. Wood (Eds.), *CCCS selected working papers 2* (pp. 753–774). Routledge.
Carlisle, C., Baker, G. A., Riley, M., & Dewey, M. (1994). Stress in midwifery: A comparison of midwives and nurses using the work environment scale. *International Journal of Nursing Studies, 31*(1), 13–22. https://doi.org/10.1016/0020-7489(94)90003-5
Castañeda, D., & Burns-Glover, A. L. (2008). *Women's friendships and romantic relationships: Culture, sexuality, and lifespan contexts*. Psychology of Women: A Handbook of Issues and Theories, 332-352.
Dill, B. T. (1983). Race, class, and gender: Prospects for an all-inclusive sisterhood. *Feminist Studies, 9*(1), 131–150.
Dubois, S., & Loisell, C. G. (2009). Cancer informational support and health care service use among individuals newly diagnosed: A mixed method approach. *Journal of Evaluation in Clinical Practice, 15*, 346–359. https://doi.org/10.1111/j.1365-2753.2008.01013.x
Floyd-Thomas, S., & Gillman, L. (2005). "The whole story is what I'm after": Womanist revolutions and liberation feminist revelations through biomythography and emancipatory historiography. *Black Theology, 3*(2), 176–199.
Fox-Genovese, E. (1979). *The personal is not political enough*. Cliomar Corporation.
Greif, G. L., & Sharpe, T. L. (2010). The friendships of women: Are there differences between African Americans and whites? *Journal of Human Behavior in the Social Environment, 20*(6), 791–807. https://doi.org/10.1080/10911351003751892
Hanasono, L. K., & Yang, F. (2016). Computer-mediated coping: Exploring the quality of supportive communication in an online discussion forum for individuals who are coping with racial discrimination. *Communication Quarterly*, 1–21. https://doi.org/10.1080/0146337 3.2015.1103292

Hochschild, A. R. (1979). Emotion work, feeling rules, and social structure. *American Journal of Sociology, 85*(3), 551–575. https://doi.org/10.1086/227049

Hochschild, A. (1983). Comment on Kemper's "social constructionist and positivist approaches to the sociology of emotions". *American Journal of Sociology, 89*(2), 432–434. https://doi.org/10.1086/227874

Hochschild, A. R. (2000). Global care chains and emotional surplus value. In A. Giddens & W. Hutton (Eds.), *On the edge: Living with global capitalism* (pp. 130–146). Jonathan Cape.

Hodnett, E. D., Gates, S., Hofmeyr, G. J., & Sakala, C. (2007). Continuous support for women during childbirth. *Cochrane Database of Systematic Reviews, 7*. Retrieved from http://www.european-doula-network.org/media/studies/Chocrane%20continuous%20support.pdf

Hooks, B. (1986). Sisterhood: Political solidarity between women. *Feminist Review, 23*, 125–138. https://doi.org/10.2307/1394725

Hunter, B. (2001). Emotion work in midwifery: A review of current knowledge. *Journal of Advanced Nursing, 34*(4), 436–444. https://doi.org/10.1046/j.1365-2648.2001.01772.x.

Husband, B. P. (2015). *The ties that bind us in sisterhood* (Doctoral Dissertation). Retrieved from ProQuest.

Institute of Medicine (US) Committee on Health and Behavior: Research, Practice, and Policy. (2001). *Health and behavior: The interplay of biological, behavioral, and societal influences*. National Academies Press. Retrieved from https://www.ncbi.nlm.nih.gov/books/NBK43749/

James, N. (1989). Emotional labour: Skill and work in the social regulation of feelings. *The Sociological Review, 37*(1), 15–42. https://doi.org/10.1111/j.1467-954X.1989.tb00019.x

James, N. (1992). Care= Organisation+ physical labour+ emotional labour. *Sociology of Health & Illness, 14*(4), 488–509.

John, V., & Parsons, E. (2006). Shadow work in midwifery: Unseen and unrecognised emotional labour. *British Journal of Midwifery, 14*(5), 266–271. https://doi.org/10.12968/bjom.2006.14.5.21046

Jones, S. M., & Wirtz, J. G. (2006). How does the comforting process work? An empirical test of an appraisal-based model of comforting. *Human Communication Research, 32*(3), 217–243.

Li, H. J. (2010). *The women's movements and the gendering of Taiwanese democracy, 1949 1999* (Doctoral dissertation). Retrieved from ProQuest.

MacGeorge, E. L., Feng, B., & Burleson, B. R. (2011). Supportive communication. In M. L. Knapp & J. A. Daly (Eds.), *Handbook of interpersonal communication* (pp. 317–354). Sage Publications.

McCubbin, H. I., & Patterson, J. M. (1983). The family stress process: The double ABCX model of adjustment and adaptation. *Marriage & Family Review, 6*(1-2), 7–37.

Morgan, R. (1970). *Sisterhood is powerful an anthology of writings from the Women's liberation movement* (1st ed.). Random House.

Morton, C. H., & Clift, E. (2014). *Birth ambassadors: Doulas and the re-emergence of woman-supported birth America*. Praeclarus Press, LLC.

Myers, S. A., & Kennedy-Lightsey, C. D. (2015). Communication in adult sibling relationships. In L. H. Turner & R. West (Eds.), *The sage handbook of family communication* (pp. 220–234). Sage Publications.

Naiman-Sessions, M., Henley, M. M., & Roth, L. M. (2017). Bearing the burden of care: Emotional burnout among maternity support workers. In *Health and health care concerns among women and racial and ethnic minorities* (pp. 99–125). Emerald Publishing Limited. https://doi.org/10.1108/S0275-495920170000035006

Netuveli, G., Wiggins, R., Hilden, Z., Montgomery, S., & Blaine, D. (2006). Quality of life at older ages: Evidence from the English longitudinal study of aging (wave 1). *Journal of Epidemiology and Community Health, 60*, 357–363.

Pascoe, E. A., & Smart Richman, L. (2009). Perceived discrimination and health: A meta-analytic review. *Psychological Bulletin, 135*(4), 531.

Peirce, C. S. (1958). *Values in a universe of chance: Selected writings of Charles Sanders Peirce*. Doubleday.

Putnam, R. D. (2001). *Bowling alone: The collapse and revival of American community*. New York, London, & Toronto: Simon & Schuster Paperbacks.

Qi, T. (2010). Transforming sisterhood to an all-relational solidarity. *Race, Gender & Class, 17*(3/4), 327–335.

Ramos, B. M. (2012). Psychosocial stress, social inequality, and mental health in Puerto Rican women in upstate New York. *Centro Journal, 24*(2), 48–67.

Remmers, H., Holtgräwe, M., & Pinkert, C. (2010). Stress and nursing care needs of women with breast cancer during primary treatment: A qualitative study. *European Journal of Oncology Nursing, 14*(1), 11–16.

Samter, W. (2003). Friendship interaction skills across the life span. In J. O. Greene & B. R. Burleson (Eds.), *Handbook of communication and social interaction skills* (pp. 637–684). Erlbaum.

Shumaker, S. A., & Brownell, A. (1984). Toward a theory of social support: Closing conceptual gaps. *Journal of Social Issues, 40*(4), 11–36.

Simmonds, F. N. (1997). Who are the sisters? Difference, feminism, and friendship. In M. Ang-Lygate, C. Corrin, M. S. Henry, & Women's Studies Network (Eds.), *Desperately seeking sisterhood: Still challenging and building* (pp. 19–30). Taylor & Francis.

Son, J., Yarnal, C., & Kerstetter, D. (2010). Engendering social capital through a leisure club for middle-aged and older women: Implications for individual and community health and Well-being. *Leisure Studies, 29*(1), 67–83. https://doi.org/10.1080/02614360903242578

Stana, A., & Flynn, M. A. (2012). Social support in a men's online eating disorder forum. *International Journal of Men's Health, 11*(2), 150–169.

Tatum, R. M. (2017). *Spirit, soul, sisterhood: Race, religion, and childbirth in New Mexico, 1900-1950* (Doctoral Dissertation). Union theological seminary in the City of New York, NY. Retrieved from ProQuest.

Toto, R. L., Man, L., Blatt, B., Simmens, S. J., & Greenberg, L. (2015). Do empathy, perspective-taking, sense of power and personality differ across undergraduate education and are they inter-related? *Advances in Health Sciences Education, 20*(1), 23–31. https://doi.org/10.1007/s10459-014-9502-z

Umberson, D., & Montez, J. K. (2010). Social relationships and health: A flashpoint for health policy. *Journal of Health and Social Behavior, 51*(1_suppl), S54–S66. https://doi.org/10.1177/0022146510383501

Verderber, K. S., & MacGeorge, E. L. (2016). *Inter-act: Interpersonal communication concepts, skills, and contexts* (14th ed.). Oxford University Press.

Whaley, D. E. (2010). *Disciplining women: Alpha kappa alpha, black counterpublics, and the cultural politics of black sororities*. SUNY Press.

Chapter 4
Medical Procedures and Discourses Around Women's Bodies

In this chapter, I analyze themes that emerged from the interviews that reveal medical perspectives on childbirth as well as themes that reveal advocacy and support for natural birth.[1] Following Chap. 2's analysis of the motivations for women to work as doulas, and also following Chap. 3's analysis of sisterhood relationships among doulas and mothers, this chapter focuses on the study participants' understandings of doula-attended childbirth in China. Many of the Chinese doulas who participated in this study expressed their advocacy for natural birth, and they strongly believed that doula-attended childbirth was associated with an increase in natural delivery. Linked to advocacy for natural birth, many doulas in this study (especially doulas coming from non-medical backgrounds) stated their critical insights about the use of epidural analgesia as a means of pain management for women in childbirth.

Globally, medical interventions during labor may include cesarean section (hereafter C-section), induced labor, use of an epidural for pain management, and electronic fetal monitoring (Hunter & Hurst, 2016). Participants revealed a common understanding of "natural childbirth" as a birthing process that did not rely on technological and medical intervention. The natural childbirth process, according to the interviews, includes spontaneous childbirth experience of labor without interventions, such as anesthesia, and a vaginal delivery. In American clinical practices, some professionals define natural birth as childbirth without medical interventions (Brubaker & Dillaway, 2009; Mansfield, 2008). Other professionals define natural birth as hospital births without usage of an epidural for pain management (Lothian, 2000; Simkin & Bolding, 2004).

---

[1] The term 自然分娩 (*zi ran fen mian* in Chinese) translates as natural birth linguistically. Moreover, interviewees in this project used the term "natural birth." Therefore, I also use the term "natural birth" in this chapter.

Z. Z. Dai, *Maternal Healthcare and Doulas in China*,
https://doi.org/10.1007/978-3-030-46963-4_4

47

Medical Procedures: Natural Birth

Several of the Chinese doulas that I interviewed associated doula-attended childbirths with natural birth. This kind of belief came from their personal experiences as they were attending expectant mothers during childbirth, from reading related articles on doula care studies, or from attending doula or childbirth education seminars. Liu Ying, an obstetrician and a doula, said,

> I think doula support childbirth is more likely to lead to a natural delivery. In my experience, doulas provide emotional and physical support for pregnant women.

Liu Ying also believed that doulas establish a relationship of trust with expectant mothers, and "the power of trust absolutely would lead pregnant women to have a natural delivery." He Pei, an obstetrician and a doula, also said,

> Doulas lead pregnant women to choose natural delivery. Although I did not conduct any research on this topic, many health scholars have proved that doulas attending laboring would increase natural delivery and reduce C-section. I have read some articles from Barbara's (Barbara Harper) seminar.

Further, some doulas I interviewed mentioned that those choosing to have a natural delivery tended to be more liberal in their beliefs about women and their bodies. Those espousing such liberal beliefs encourage women to be in rhythm with their bodies during child labor and to move freely in response to what they feel in terms of movement and positions (Lamaze International, 2018). These were referred to as "liberal positions" in childbirth by the interviewees. These movements (e.g., sitting, walking, squatting) of the pregnant body are considered helpful for moving the baby through the pelvis and enlarging pelvic diameters. Jiang Min, a doula and lactation consultant, elaborated her experience with liberal positions in labor, which she learned from the Lamaze Childbirth Education seminar. Jiang Min said,

> I taught one of the mothers about liberal [body] positions, and she walked around in the delivery room when she felt a contraction. She also squatted several times, which enlarged the pelvis diameter. She believed that her body naturally could find a comfortable position to deliver the baby. I remembered that her delivery was not long, and she felt good. In my opinion, my attendance of her laboring supported her belief in natural birth.

In addition to liberal body positions and free movements, some doulas have suggested the use of a yoga ball could be helpful for women in labor. Jiang Min indicated that since 2015 all the pre-delivery rooms and labor suites in the maternal hospital she worked for had "at least one yoga ball." Qin Nan, an obstetrician and doula, also said she liked to introduce a yoga ball or peanut ball to women in labor: "Women can sit on the yoga ball, and the 'sit-down' position will enlarge pelvic diameters."

Su Yi, an obstetrician and doula, admitted that some strategies of doula care were very helpful for expectant mothers in labor suites. These helpful strategies included massages that could reduce the women's pain, and small talk between obstetricians and expectant mothers that served to reduce their stress and anxiety. Unlike other doulas who held positive attitudes toward doula-attended childbirth, Su Yi expressed some concerns regarding doula care in Chinese maternal hospitals. She was particularly concerned about how the doulas promoted natural birth and liberal positions exclusively. She said,

> Many American childbirth educators talked about natural birth, liberal position as well as non-medical intervention. However, Americans are different from Chinese. In the U.S., it is normal to see a newborn baby at about 4,500 grams or even heavier. In China, a baby like that is overweight. Moreover, the size of an American woman's pelvis is larger than a Chinese woman's. Also, women's body weights are different among American and Chinese women. These fundamental differences were not emphasized in the doula care seminars, which were quite important.

Su Yi's observations on the differences between Chinese and American women's bodies are important to point out. On one hand, Chinese doulas use an American/Western disciplinary control mechanism to replace the Chinese patriarchal and government dominance because it claims to privilege women's bodies. On the other hand, it does not recognize that not all women's bodies are the same, which creates a different hierarchy regarding knowledge and epistemology.

Su Yi also commented that Chinese obstetricians, midwives, and Chinese doulas should not listen to and apply everything that American physicians or childbirth educators had taught them. The point that Su Yi raised resonates with transnational, postcolonial, and black feminist critiques of white/liberal and Western feminism. As Chandra Mohanty (1988) notes in her work *Under Western Eyes: Feminist Scholarship and Colonial Discourse*,

> For in the context of a first/third-world balance of power, feminist analyses which perpetrate and sustain the hegemony of the idea of the superiority of the West produce a corresponding set of universal images of the "third-world woman," images like the veiled woman, the powerful mother, the chaste virgin, the obedient wife, etc. These images exist in universal ahistorical splendor, setting in motion a colonialist discourse which exercises a very specific power in defining, coding and maintaining existing first/third-world connections. (p. 81)

It is clear that in this health communication context the adoption of a Westernized model of the doula care system creates a different kind of power dynamic and does not always epistemically privilege the Chinese woman's rights to decision making over her own body, nor does it cater to the holistic well-being of the Chinese woman.

Huang Ru, another of my interviewees, became a doula when she was pregnant with her first baby. Coming from a non-medical background, Ru voiced her concerns about the promotion of doulas and doula care in China. She said,

> I know there is a large number of Chinese pregnant women who intend to pursue pure natural birth because they think it is beautiful and empowered, but they do not know whether these are suitable for them or not. Some doulas directly introduce American childbirth models to Chinese pregnant women (e.g., laboring in the forest), which is very irresponsible. These kinds of doulas just want to brainwash Chinese pregnant women. We should not be polarized nor extreme.

Huang Ru's critiques on the promotion of doula care in China reflect Rosalind Gill's (2008) work *Culture and Subjectivity in Neoliberal and Postfeminist Times*, in which Gill discusses what happens through "adoption of these models in a neoliberal model of individual choice." Gill writes,

> In the desire to "respect" girls "choices" any notion of cultural influence seems to have been evacuated entirely. Yet how can we account for the dominance of a fashion item such as a g-string without any reference to culture? … Yet one of the problems with this focus on autonomous choices is that it remains complicit with, rather than critical of, postfeminist and neoliberal discourses that see individuals as entrepreneurial actors who are rational, calculating and self-regulating. The neoliberal subject is required to bear full responsibility for their life biography no matter how severe the constraints upon their action. (p. 446, p. 447)

Similar to Huang Ru's statements, Yue Le—an experienced midwife—stated that some Chinese doulas and pregnant women adopt extreme forms of natural birth. Yue Le said,

> They are being brainwashed. It is empowering to listen to their bodies. However, do they really listen to their bodies? Or do they just listen to the polarized ideas of pursuing a natural birth?

Yue Le also added one case from her professional experiences,

> A mother's water was broken for more than four days. We (obstetricians and midwives) suggested she choose C-section due to her extreme case, based on medical considerations, but she still insisted on natural birth. We wanted to make sure both she and her child were safe. Also, she was exhausted and almost did not have energy to push during child labor. At the end, she did have a C-section. The baby was sent to the newborn's room immediately for critical healthcare. Pediatricians found that the child's skull was extruded due to the long-labor process. Being an obstetrics staff member, I did not encourage the expectant mother to have a C-section. However, it is necessary to have medical intervention or technical intervention in some extreme cases. I believe all the obstetrics staff are helping pregnant women rather than hurting them. The stubborn belief in natural birth is not right.

Yet, even as they criticized strong faith in natural childbirth that in their view was problematically adopted—meaning, not adapted to the specifics of a Chinese woman's body—several doulas also voiced their concerns regarding the use of pharmacological pain relief technologies. In particular, they were concerned about the use of epidural analgesia in labor. In the discourse of natural childbirth, the use of an epidural is considered a form of medical intervention. He Pei, an obstetrician and a doula, shared one of her cases with a birthing mother:

> We used yoga ball at the first birthing stage, and it helped her to relax. We worked very well. She did not use epidural or any types of medical intervention as pain management methods. We had conversations on the topic of epidural several times before her labor. She trusted me, and she was very confident in natural delivery without using epidural.

Epidural analgesia is the most common technique for labor pain management (Zhang & Ren, 2017) and is defined as one method of medical intervention (Lamaze International, 2018; Newnham et al., 2016). The use of epidural analgesia is very high in the United States and many other Western countries (Pregnancy and birth, 2018; Silva & Halpen, 2010). However, the use of epidural analgesia as a pain management method accounts for less than 7% of all deliveries in China (Wang & Li, 2017). Ling-Qun Hu and her colleagues note in their studies that many Chinese women do not currently have the option of an epidural (2016). In Chinese clinics, some midwives and obstetricians called a natural delivery with use of epidural as a pain-free delivery or painless labor (*wu tong fen mian* in Chinese). Some Chinese doulas in this study were critical about the usage of an epidural for labor pain management. He Pei, for instance, notes,

> I would not say I am against epidural labor analgesia as well as spinal painkiller. However, I think the usage of epidural labor analgesia for women in labor should be carefully reviewed and evaluated. In my opinion, only a few women in labor warrant response of "must use epidural" since the pain in laboring is more physiological rather than pathological.

Jian Ning, a doula and lactation consultant, observed that epidural analgesia has become, in her words, a "super star" in the delivery room. It became common belief that this procedure could save every woman from suffering the labor pains. In her opinion, many obstetrics staff have misused the epidural. Jian Ning said,

> In fact, only a few women may really need to use an epidural in labor as pain management. The seminar I took with International Childbirth Education Association (hereafter ICEA) informed me about the negative impacts of using an epidural. It is a medical intervention, and we should stop using it.

Jian Ning learned about epidural analgesia from ICEA seminars; likewise, Lin Jing received related information about epidural analgesia from ICEA courses she took in 2016. Lin Jing also considered the epidural to be a medical intervention. She believed that a natural delivery should not include the use of unnecessary medical interventions—and she included epidural analgesia as one such unnecessary medical intervention. Recalling her experiences, Lin Jing revealed that there was a commercial promotion of epidural analgesia for use in the delivery room by midwives and obstetricians. She said,

> I used to work as a doula in one private hospital. The obstetrics staff members informed me that more than 95% of the expectant mothers received epidural analgesia during the laboring process in this hospital. I got a sense that obstetrics staff encourage and then force them to receive an epidural, which is unnecessary. Thus, I think expectant mothers need to have an ability to distinguish the information or advice they receive from obstetrics staff. I remember that one mother asked a midwife what some pros and cons were for receiving an epidural, and the midwife answered, "all the pregnant women use it, and you should too." I think the midwife did not tell the truth to the mother. Moreover, the usage of epidural analgesia has become a commercial action, which midwives and obstetricians promote to every woman in labor. If a mother eventually chooses to use an epidural, that is fine, and it is her choice. However, if most of the obstetrics staff promote or advocate for using epidural, I think it is not right.

Shen Yu, a hospital-based doula, also shared a similar opinion about using epidural analgesia. She said that she never encouraged expectant mothers to use epidural analgesia during labor, although she always informed them about the pros and cons of an epidural. She insisted that every woman should make the decision (to use an epidural or not) by herself. However, the reality was that many midwives and obstetricians were promoting the usage of epidural analgesia in labor since they received extra money to do so. Thus, Shen Yu believed that the use of epidural analgesia in China had become a commercial practice among midwives and obstetricians.

Love What I Doula For: Doula's Belief

This chapter focuses on participants' understandings of doula-attended childbirth in China. Doula care has introduced the discourse of natural childbirth and the use of epidural analgesic as pain management. Some doulas expressed their beliefs that doula-attended childbirth is associated with an increasing rate of natural delivery, which they believe is healthier for women's bodies. On the contrary, some doulas in this study voiced their concerns on the adoption of a Westernized model of the doula care system, which creates a contradictory situation in the labor suite.

Many of the Chinese doulas I interviewed voiced a strong belief that doula support during childbirth increased the rate of natural births. Natural birthing was considered to be healthy for women in general. On one hand, the Chinese doulas who had no medical training noted that they learned about the connection between doula-attended childbirth and natural birth from different childbirth education seminars or doula training programs. As Huang Ru, one of the doulas with no medical background said, "I learned that natural birth (as a delivery method) was better than C-section from ICEA seminars." In other words, some of the doulas received information about natural births as secondhand knowledge. On the other hand, some of the doulas with no medical background believed that natural delivery was healthy and more beneficial than C-section due to their personal labor experiences. Thus, some doulas learned about the benefits of natural birth through training offered within medical settings and other doulas learned about the benefits of natural birth through embodied experience. Jian Ning compared the difference in her learning about childbirth labor since she had the opportunity to have both a medicalized experience and a natural birth experience. These were two different kinds of experience. Her first delivery included induction followed by a C-section, and her second delivery was a natural delivery. Based on her comparison of her own experience in both settings, Jian Nan was able to understand the difference through embodied knowledge. Therefore, when she did receive training from ICEA and other doula care organizations, as she worked toward being a doula, the discussions from these seminars only reinforced her experience-based belief that natural birth without the use of an epidural was the better delivery method for women in general.

In the case of doulas from medical backgrounds (e.g., He Pei, Liu Ying), their medical school training had taught them that natural birth was a much better choice for women from an evidence-based medical perspective. Thus, the epistemic conditions of learning that natural birth is a better process were different in this case than in the case of the doula with no prior medial training and background. He Pei made statements such as "the agony of natural birth would increase a mother's bond with her child," "natural birth would give a good beginning for breastfeeding," and "woman's body would recover from labor faster than from C-section."

Both He Pei and Jian Ning held positive attitudes toward natural birth, but they had different languages for the procedures of natural birth. Before they moved toward doula care and childbirth education as their major careers, they had received different levels of training on childbirth and medical science in general. He Pei and

Jian Ning had different epistemic conditions of learning—those conditions led them to a different experiential understanding of childbirth necessary for how they view natural birth.

In 2015, the World Health Organization reported that 46 percent of Chinese babies were delivered by C-section rather than vaginal birth (Ji et al., 2015; McNeil Jr., 2017). There were two reasons for the high percentage of C-section in China. On one hand, many parents and grandparents demanded C-section to assure that births took place on an auspicious day as marked in the astrological calendar or because the family members believed that a surgically removed infant was more likely to be perfectly formed. Chinese parents were also opting for C-section to ensure a preferred school admission because the Chinese educational system regards a birth date of August 31 as the last date for entrance-level admission to elementary school. Children born in the remaining 4 months of the year were delayed elementary school admission by 1 year.

Through the interviews I conducted, the overall role of doulas seems to be that of birth educators for Chinese parents. The doulas help expectant parents understand the pros and cons of natural delivery and C-sections, respectively. Doulas believe that it is important to point out that Chinese women should not be forced to choose C-sections as their delivery methods because their families wanted to pick a delivery date or because the government has scheduled school admission dates for their children. Along with cultural beliefs about family decision making and China's national plan for children's education, pressure to choose C-section has been a burden on women, their bodies, and their reproductive rights—or as Foucault (1979) stated, "discipline."

Contradictions

As I explained in the previous chapters, medical science and authoritative physicians (including both obstetricians and midwives) devalue or even pathologize women's bodies and bodily process, and women have been excluded from existing medical information and from making decisions about their own bodies (Wong, n.d.; Bornstein & Emler, 2001; Dalmiya & Alcoff, 1993; Parry, 2008; Vlassoff, 2007). Thus, women's bodily experiences were excluded from routine medical decision-making processes. Approaching the question of "which type of laboring method should I use," an obstetrician's authoritative response would be considered from a medical science perspective, with a communicative approach like, "Let me tell you this. To make sure both you and the baby are safe, I suggest you choose...." Given the ratio of obstetrics staff (physicians, nurses, midwives) to patients (pregnant women) in China, it was understandable that doctors carried heavy burdens in the work. There was no doubt about their dedication, professionalism, and being highly responsible for their patients. However, the communicative approach was not very effective nor approachable. Through the interviews I had with doulas, several interviewees informed me that they sometimes observed these types of conversations. Some obstetricians approached pregnant women with a kind of firm, authoritative, scientific tone that left little room for negotiation or discussion. Lin Ning shared her observations when she recalled one of her first labor experiences:

> Being a pregnant woman in labor, you just lay down on the bed in the delivery room and wait to "labor." You would be half- (sometimes fully) naked in front of obstetricians and midwives who are (or might be) strangers. However, I feel that no one (or rarely someone) cares what you think. No one really cares about your thoughts about body-shame or anything else.

Although obstetricians (along with midwives) propose their medical decisions as "suggestions," many pregnant women tend to interpret such suggestions as confirmed decisions. As Morgan (1998) states, "Once again, and over and over, women are first medically conceptualized and then 'diagnosed' as naturally sickly, blamed for being sick, treated as sick, and seen as irrationally pathogenic by nature" (p. 103). Women's pregnancy, defined as a diseased condition, routinely requires medical "treatment" in order to be cured and healed (Treichler, 1990).

The culture of doula care has emerged as a women-centered response to the medicalization of women's bodies and bodily processes, as well as a means to advocate natural childbirth (Dwyer, 2012; Papagni & Buckner, 2006). Therefore, the emerging discourses of doulas and doula care for women's childbirth experiences have been positioned challenging the scientific knowledge and medical technologies that have dominated women's bodies (Campbell-Voytal et al., 2011; Shaw, 2013).

However, the doula care system is feeding into a new type of possible state control on women's body. It is a paradigm shift but not necessarily a shift that favors women's autonomy for choice, even though it seems that the doulas themselves—the ones I interviewed at least—struggle with the ethics around issues of decisions and choices. Some Chinese doulas produce hierarchies where the pregnant women's bodies are still subject to power and structures—even as there is a shift in the processes and methods for child birthing. Thus, when a doula encourages a pregnant woman to pursue natural birth without truly considering the woman's bodily situation, she is not giving enough information to the pregnant mother so that she may make her own decisions on what options she might pursue for her own and her offspring's well-being. In those situations, I do not see a difference between "empowered doulas" and "authoritative obstetrician/midwives." Even if the doulas may be empowered, the pregnant woman giving birth is still objectified—and the options for her to exert her agency in decision making are not that much better in one instance or the other. It remains to be seen, however, whether the shift to doula mediation in childbirth practices will be incorporated into Chinese governmentality around the Chinese women's pregnancy and bodily autonomy.

Huang Ru and Yue Le perceived polarization within the discourse of natural birth and birth assisted with medical interventions. Natural birth for many pregnant Chinese women may not be feasible, and when some doulas advocate too strongly for natural birth, they may adopt an obstetrician's authority. Thus, some doulas reinforce the "authoritative knowledge of natural birth" in their relationships with pregnant women. This type of doula care does not empower pregnant women to recognize or embrace their agency during labor. Having a natural delivery over C-section does not automatically empower women or remove them from the medical system's disciplining influence. Furthermore, women should not be shamed through such statements as "you made a mistake because you did not deliver your child naturally through vaginal birth."

Thus, I suggest that the fundamental arguments are not about whether women should choose natural birth or C-section or whether women should have a vaginal birth without medical and technological interventions. Instead, "choice" is central to the childbirth discourse, and decisions about childbirth should be made by the expectant mother herself. As I discussed in Chap. 1, the power of obstetrics staff (physicians, midwives, nurses) is their authority to determine what counts as legitimate knowledge about childbirth. Therefore, I suggest that an expectant mother's decision to undergo natural birth or a C-section should not be dominated by an obstetrician or a midwife, both of whom gained scientific knowledge and training through medical schools; and neither should the mother's decision be controlled by a doula, who was educated by Western/American childbirth organizations and who speaks with "authoritative knowledge" (Davis-Floyd et al., 2009; Jordan & Davis-Floyd, 1993; Henley, 2015). I also suggest that the "choice" of childbirth is about women's agency and autonomy. A doula's purpose is to "help [a] woman have a safe and satisfying childbirth as the woman defines it. It [is] not the role of the doula to discourage the mother from her choice" (DONA, 2021). A doula's role is to help women become informed about their options, including explaining the risks and benefits of different delivery methods and of using different medical/technological interventions. Doulas thus could play a unique role in a woman's labor process because they were employed by pregnant women but have no decision-making rights and responsibilities.

Importantly, natural birth should not be the only birth choice for women. It is beneficial for expectant mothers to receive emotional, informational, and physical support from doulas. As I explained in Chap. 1, the One-Child Policy is ended, and all legally married couples are permitted to have a second child. Under the Second-Child Policy, a growing number of Chinese families expect women to have two children. One study participant even said, "Once a woman labored the first child through natural birth, she could start to prepare to get pregnant for her second child in a month." In my training at WeCare WMH, I heard a doula and a midwife talk about the idea of having a second child with a woman who had just finished labor. The midwife said to the woman, "You had an enjoyable labor experience, right? Look at how cute your baby is." Then the doula added:

> You could start to think and prepare for the second one sooner or later. If you had a C-section, you would not able to do that for one or two years. But with natural delivery, you can. I would like to serve as your doula again.

This chapter focused on Chinese doulas' perceptions of doula-attended childbirth and their understandings of the shifts in medical practices resulting from the interventions made by doulas—specifically, the value of natural childbirth and the use of epidural analgesia as pain management. Many doulas in this study described their advocacy for natural birth, and they strongly believed that doula-attended childbirth (or when pregnant women received doula care) was associated with increased rates of natural delivery. Participants' responses suggest that the doula care profession has created space for pregnant women to make decisions and choices about childbirth by themselves, thereby empowering women. From a women-centered health communication point of view, not only would their advocacy and care work reject the perception of authoritative, medical knowledge, but it would also represent a rejection of the medicalization of women's bodies. As I have suggested, it is also necessary to encourage women to have resilience and to understand the strengths and limitations of natural birth, as well as medical and technological interventions for childbirth.

References

Bornstein, B. H., & Emler, A. C. (2001). Rationality in medical decision making: a review of the literature on doctors' decision-making biases. *Journal of Evaluation in Clinical Practice, 7*(2), 97–107.

Brubaker, S. J., & Dillaway, H. E. (2009). Medicalization, natural childbirth and birthing experiences. *Sociology Compass, 3*(1), 31–48. https://doi.org/10.1111/j.1751-9020.2008.00183.x

Campbell-Voytal, K., McComish, J., Visger, J., Rowland, C., & Kelleher, J. (2011). Postpartum doulas: Motivations and perceptions of practice. *Midwifery, 27*(6), E214–E221. https://doi.org/10.1016/j.midw.2010.09.006

Davis-Floyd, R. E., & Cheyney, M. (2009). Birth and the big bad wolf: an evolutionary perspective. In H. Selin & P. K. Stone (Eds.), *Childbirth across cultures* (pp.1–22). Dordrecht, Heidelberg, London, & New York: Springer.

Dalmiya, V., & Alcoff, L. (1993). Are "old wives' tales" justified? In L. Alcoff & E. Potter (Eds.), *Feminist Epistemology* (pp. 217–244). Routledge.

DONA International, (n.d.). About DONA International. Retrieved November 5, 2021, from https://www.dona.org/the-dona-advantage/about/

Dwyer, J. (2012). *Continuums of reproductive choice: Theorizing doula care* (Master Thesis). Carleton University, Ottawa, Canada. Retrieved from ProQuest.

Foucault, M. (1979). *Discipline and punish: The birth of the prison* (translated from French by Alan Sheridan). New York: Vintage Books.

Gill, R. (2008). Culture and subjectivity in neoliberal and postfeminist times. *Subjectivity, 25*(1), 432–445. https://doi.org/10.1057/sub.2008.28

Henley, M. M. (2015). Alternative and authoritative knowledge: The role of certification for defining expertise among doulas. *Social Currents, 2*(3), 260–279. https://doi.org/10.1177/2329496515589851

Hu, L., Flood, P., Li, Y., Tao, W., Zhao, P., Xia, Y., … Wong, C. (2016). No pain labor & delivery: A global health initiative's impact on clinical outcomes in China. *Anesthesia and Analgesia, 122*(6), 1931–1938. https://doi.org/10.1213/ANE.0000000000001328

Hunter, C. A., & Hurst, A. (2016). *Understanding doulas and childbirth: Women, love, and advocacy*. Palgrave Macmillan. https://doi.org/10.1057/978-1-137-48,536-6

Ji, H., Jiang, H., Yang, L., Qian, X., & Tang, S. (2015). Factors contributing to the rapid rise of caesarean section: A prospective study of primiparous Chinese women in shanghai. *BMJ Open, 5*(11), e008994. https://doi.org/10.1136/bmjopen-2015-008994

Jordan, B., & Davis-Floyd, R. (1993). *Birth in four cultures: A crosscultural investigation of childbirth in Yucatan.* Holland, Sweden, and the United States. Long Grove, Illinois: Waveland Press.

Lamaze International. (2018). *Labor positions: Position statement.* Washington, DC. Retrieved from https://www.lamaze.org/laborpositions

Lothian, J. A. (2000). Why natural childbirth? *The Journal of Perinatal Education, 9*(4), 44–46. https://doi.org/10.1624/105812400X87905

Mansfield, B. (2008). The social nature of natural childbirth. *Social Science & Medicine, 66*(5).

McNeil Jr., D. (2017). Study finds lower, but still high, rate of C-sections in China. *New York Times (Online).* Retrieved from https://www.nytimes.com/2017/01/09/health/c-sectionbirths-china.html

Mohanty, C. T. (1988). Under western eyes: Feminist scholarship and colonial discourses. *Feminist Review, 30*(1), 61–88. https://doi.org/10.1057/fr.1988.42

Morgan, K. P. (1998). Contested Bodies, Contested Knowledges: Women, Health, and politics of Medicalization. In S. Sherwin (Ed.), *The politics of women's health: Exploring agency and autonomy* (pp. 83–121). Temple University Press.

Newnham, E. C., Pincombe, J. I., & McKellar, L. V. (2016). Critical medical anthropology in midwifery research: a framework for ethnographic analysis. *Global Qualitative Nursing Research, 3,* 1–6. https://doi.org/10.1177/2333393616675029

Papagni, K., & Buckner, E. (2006). Doula support and attitudes of intrapartum nurses: A qualitative study from the patient's perspective. *The Journal of Perinatal Education, 15*(1), 11–18. https://doi.org/10.1624/105812406X92949

Parry, D. C. (2008). "We wanted a birth experience, not a medical experience": Exploring Canadian women's use of midwifery. *Health Care for Women International, 29*(8–9), 784–806.

Pregnancy and birth: Epidural and painkillers for labor pain relief. (2018, March 22). *Informed Health Online.* Retrieved from https://www.ncbi.nlm.nih.gov/pubmedhealth/PMH0072751/

Shaw, J. (2013). The medicalization of birth and midwifery as resistance. *Health Care for Women International, 34*(6), 522–536. https://doi.org/10.1080/07399332.2012.736569

Silva, M., & Halpern, S. H. (2010). Epidural analgesia for labor: Current techniques. *Local and Regional Anesthesia, 3,* 143–153. https://doi.org/10.2147/LRA.S10237

Simkin, P., & Bolding, A. (2004). Update on nonpharmacologic approaches to relieve labor pain and prevent suffering. *Journal of Midwifery & Women's Health, 49*(6), 489–504.

Treichler, P. A. (1990). Feminism, Medicine, and the Meaning of Childbirth. In M. Jacobus, E. Keller, & S. Shuttleworth (Eds.), *Body/Politics: Women and the Discourses of Science* (pp. 129–138). Routledge.

Vlassoff, C. (2007). Gender differences in determinants and consequences of health and illness. *Journal of Health, Population, and Nutrition, 25*(1), 47. Retrieved from https://www.ncbi.nlm.nih.gov/pmc/articles/PMC3013263/

Wang, X., & Li, W. (2017, September 07). Voices rise for painless childbirth. *China Daily.* Retrieved from https://search.proquest.com/docview/1936007487?accountid=26417

Wong, Y. (n.d.). *Integrating the gender perspective in medical and health education and research.* Retrieved from http://www.un.org/womenwatch/daw/csw/integrate.htm

Zhang, W., & Ren, M. (2017). Optimal dose of epidural Dexmedetomidine added to Ropivacaine for epidural labor Analgesia: A pilot study. *Evidence-Based Complement & Alternative Medicine,* 1–4. Retrieved from https://www.ncbi.nlm.nih.gov/pubmed/28656055?dopt=Abstract

Chapter 5
Disagreement and Conflicts: Who Is in Charge of the Delivery Room?

Interpersonal conflict is defined broadly as disagreement between two interdependent people who perceive that they have incompatible goals (Guerrero et al., 2011). In this chapter, I focus on the themes that emerged from the interviews regarding conflicts. The underlying conflicts that interviewees shared stemmed from the different ways doulas and obstetricians/midwives perceived doula care and understood doula professional training.

As I explained in the previous chapters, doula care as a profession is relatively new in China, and it is introduced to Chinese clinics through American medical practices. The term "doula" in Chinese culture acquires meaning from the doula's purpose in context and is differentiated structurally from Western doulas (Cheung et al., 2005, 2009). For instance, the term "doula" denotes not only a medical profession in Chinese contexts, it also refers to a medical instrument utilized during natural birth to help women reduce pain.[1]

Conflict is inevitable in most types of relationships (Verderber & Macgeorge, 2016). In the Chinese context of doula care profession, there are conflicts between doulas and obstetricians/midwives. On one hand, relational conflicts might hurt relationships, but on the other hand, conflicts can help expose important issues and contribute to learning, creativity, trust, and openness (Brake et al., 1995). Hence, it is also important to understand how and in which directions the Chinese doula care profession develops through dialectic relational conflicts since these are also spaces where larger discursive shifts begin as meanings are contested and redefined in spaces of praxis.

Who Is in Charge?: Disagreement and Relational Conflicts

Many Chinese doulas coming from a non-medical educational background described their working experiences with obstetricians and midwives in the labor suites as "full of conflicts and misunderstandings." Xue Meimei has worked with several maternal hospitals (mainly private hospitals) and served as a private doula for

---

[1] As I noted in the previous chapter, Wang Wei, one of the interviewees, observed that one mom delivered a baby next to her using a doula equipment.

© The Author(s), under exclusive license to Springer Nature Switzerland AG 2021
Z. Z. Dai, *Maternal Healthcare and Doulas in China*,
https://doi.org/10.1007/978-3-030-46963-4_5

various expectant mothers for more than two years. In her interviews, she shared the following experience working in a delivery room. Xue Meimei said,

> For instance, I explained the pros and cons of oxytocin to an expectant mother. Then the expectant mother denied the suggestion of receiving oxytocin from the obstetricians. At that moment, I could tell obstetricians were very unhappy. When this kind of small conflict occurred, it brought some challenges for me to work with the same group of obstetrics staff in the future.

Xue Meimei also mentioned that some obstetricians directly said to her that they "hoped this kind of misunderstanding would not occur again." In fact, Xue Meimei interpreted the statement to mean that she should not disagree with obstetricians' medical decisions in the future, and that she should not provide any suggestions to the expectant mother. She added,

> I have realized that they might not welcome me to work as a doula in the delivery room next time. I was very frustrated. I tried to avoid this kind of conflicts with obstetrics staff in the labor suites. Sometimes, I had to apologize to them afterwards in order to maintain a good relationship with them.

Meimei apologized for the conflict, and many other doulas in this study also mentioned they had apologized to obstetricians and midwives for conflicts. Although sometimes doulas internally thought it was not "their fault," they said "sorry" to repair the relationship damage caused by the conflicts that had occurred in the labor suites.

In another case, Shen Yu, a hospital doula coming from a non-medical background, voiced her concerns about midwives and obstetricians who claimed to practice doula care in the delivery rooms. Shen Yu indicated that there was a growing number of obstetrics staff who believed that they had the ability to provide professional doula care for expectant mothers in the delivery rooms because they had received some form of doula training. However, Shen Yu argued that most of the obstetricians and midwives did not do great doula care work. She said,

> It is great to hear they started to use verbal language to encourage expectant mothers and comfort them. However, except verbal language, they normally do not fully practice professional doula care for pregnant women. In my opinion, there are many differences between professional doulas and obstetricians and/or midwives with doula care training, although they have participated in lots of doula care related workshops and/or seminars. These two groups of people are different. For instance, obstetricians and/or midwives would suggest expectant mothers use an epidural during labor in order to manage pain. Professional doulas would rarely do that. I learned it from some books and Tamela's (Hatcher) talks that an epidural was a medical intervention, and doulas should not suggest women to use it.

Since Shen Yu worked as a hospital-based doula, she formed coworker relationships with many obstetricians and midwives. She mentioned she always tried to avoid starting a conflict or would withdraw from a conflict with her obstetrics coworkers at the hospital. "They are in charge in the labor suite. They are more authoritative and powerful."

Compared to Xue Meimei's negative work experiences and Shen Yu's criticism of obstetricians and midwives, Lin Jing shared her positive work experiences with obstetricians and midwives. "They often welcomed me to enter in the delivery rooms," Lin Jing said. Lin Jing mentioned that before she could enter the delivery room she had to sign several legal documents for the hospitals since she was not an official hospital staff member. Lin Jing said,

When midwives knew I had labor experiences and had doula care trainings, they were very happy. They told me that I really helped them a lot in terms of providing support for women in the delivery rooms. They even told me that if each woman could have a doula with her, midwives' work would be easier and more effective.

It is important to point out that Lin Jing was the only one mother doula who described her working relationships with obstetricians and midwives in the delivery rooms as happy, welcoming, and encouraging.

Doulas who came from medical backgrounds and who worked (currently or previously) as obstetricians or midwives also expressed concern and hesitation about doulas and doula work in the delivery rooms. They expressed their concerns even though they claimed to practice doula care with pregnant women. Su Yi stated that she understood doula care and always loved to practice doula care in her clinical work. However, Su Yi added,

When I am in the delivery room, I do not allow doulas (the non-medical background doulas) to interrupt my work. By saying that, I mean doulas cannot influence the medical decision I make for the pregnant women. I had one experience in which a doula kept talking with the expectant mother all the time, which led the woman to become very tired and exhausted. It had a negative impact on the laboring process of the expectant mother.

Qin Nan suggested that the conflicts and misunderstandings between obstetrics staff (obstetricians, midwives, and nurses[2]) and non-medical background doulas were caused by "different understandings of medical knowledge and the evaluation of clinical risks." Qin Nan explained her points through her stories, and she said,

I used to work as an obstetrician, and I am working as a childbirth educator to promote doula-attended childbirth and respectful maternal health care in the hospital. It is very difficult for public hospitals in my city (a tier-two city) to allow private doulas to enter in the delivery rooms. Most of the obstetricians thought private doulas (who did not receive a medical degree) brought lots of risks to the delivery rooms. Being an obstetrician with a lot of clinical experiences, I definitely understand the meaning of the risks in labor suites. Thus, it is very hard for doulas to provide doula care for expectant mothers in labor. Meanwhile, it is impossible to ask obstetricians or midwives to only pay attention to one woman in labor. Regularly, three or four obstetrics staff are working for 20 pregnant women in a delivery room.

---

[2] Obstetricians and midwives serve as different medical roles for birthing women in the labor suites. However, doulas refer to both as obstetrics staff regarding the relational conflicts in labor suites. Therefore, in this chapter's discussion, "obstetrics staff" refers to obstetricians and midwives.

Shall We Talk?: A Communication Approach

Some of the doulas I interviewed expressed concerns about conflicts from a relational perspective. Most of the conflicts emerged from the relational interactions between doulas and obstetrics staff in labor suites. As I learned in the interviews, many Chinese doulas, like Xue Meimei, held different opinions from those of obstetrics staff regarding medical interventions (e.g., using oxytocin or practicing induction) for women in labor. Also, doulas were not satisfied with the doula support that obstetrics staff claimed to practice in women's labor. Moreover, obstetrics staff had conflicts with doulas because they sometimes viewed the doulas' work as an "interruption" of regular medical practices for women in labor, as well as "disregard for the accurate medical decisions" that they believed should be made by obstetrics staff.

What Xue Meimei's conflicts (and other doulas) point to is an epistemic struggle over the knowledge of the child birthing process. It is the same as with the conflict where obstetrics staff believe that doula work is only performative and does not involve informed practices of maternity health care that go beyond verbal communication (e.g., speaking).

Dalmiya and Alcoff (1993), in their work *Are "Old Wives' Tales" Justified,* note that the traditional epistemology has reduced women's knowledge to the status of "old wives' tales" since traditional epistemology focuses on "propositional knowledge" (p. 220). They further argue that the paradigm of knowing creates "a hierarchy of knowledges that replicates the mind/body and mental/manual hierarchies" (p. 11) or "epistemic discrimination" (p. 220). Dalmiya and Alcoff start the article by suggesting that the way current society epistemologically defines knowledge is limited and does not reveal the role of tacit and embodied knowledge. They use a story from the Indian epic *The Mahabharata* to explain their points. A dutiful wife, confined to her household duties in a patriarchal context, and assumed to be illiterate and lacking in wisdom acquired through the reading of scriptures and through meditation, presumes to tell a Brahmin—a learned sage—how to find *Truth.* Her advice to him angers the self-important Brahmin who considers himself as very powerful, having spent much time in meditation (Dalmiya & Alcoff, 1993, pp. 218–219). In one moment of ego-driven anger, the Brahmin loses all the power derived from time spent in meditation. The dutiful wife, on the other hand, reveals how her knowledge, gained through everyday experience and understanding, gives her access to wisdom far greater than that acquired by the Brahmin through extensive meditation spent away from society in pursuit of knowledge and wisdom. She reveals that in order to be learned it is not necessary to be away from one's everyday responsibilities and assume a so-called "objective" distance by staying away from one's familial obligations. This is not the same as contemporary feminist claims of the personal is political; rather, it highlights the role of processual, tacit and contextual knowledge acquisition versus knowledge acquired through a static, distanced, view-from-nowhere perspective.

Dalmiya and Alcoff connect the dutiful wife from *The Mahabharata* tale with a discussion of "old wives' tales" and explain how these tales contained embodied knowledge gained from women's own embodied experience of childbirth across generations, which was then transferred to women generationally through context-specific, embedded praxis. Dalmiya and Alcoff particularly discuss the role of midwives in the care of a woman's body. Midwives' skills were enhanced by their ability to identify and connect empathically with the expectant mothers' needs. Skill, knowledge and practice was thus transferred from generation to generation through "hearsay" rather than through "authoritative" books that collected "facts" stated as propositions (Dalmiya & Alcoff, 1993, p. 224, p. 225, p. 229; Towler & Bramall, 1986; Ehrenreich & English, 2010). However, with the increasing importance of propositional knowledge—where knowledge is reported as abstracted from a point of view, and where the experience and situated location of the knowledge producer is made invisible—these women were considered ignorant. Their knowledge was acquired through experience and revealed their point of view—they came to their understanding of the body through personal experience. Therefore, midwives came to be viewed as "ignorant, or naïve trouble makers," and their knowledge about childbearing, rearing, and herbal medicines began to be denigrated as mere belief and superstition. They were "considered to be mere tales or unscientific hearsay and fail[ed] to get accorded the honorific status of knowledge" (Dalmiya & Alcoff, 1993, p. 217). In other words, the "old wives/midwives" who possessed contextual knowledge about maternity were cast as "backward, ignorant, or naïve trouble makers" in an alternative knowledge system (Jordan & Davis-Floyd, 1993, p. 152; Dalmiya & Alcoff, 1993, p. 217).

From this project, I learned that some women started to move toward doula care profession and childbirth education as their careers during and/or after their own pregnancies. In other words, doulas utilize their embodied knowledge for women in the child birthing process. Therefore, the rejection of doulas (or devaluation of doula care work) by some obstetrics staff in some current maternity labor suites is based on an epistemology that privileges propositional knowledge[3] and does not reveal the role of women's embodied knowledge. A contestation over the process exists on both sides, obstetric staff and doulas, and the war of positions is not clear cut—the struggle over what counts as knowledge of women's bodies and childbirth caregiving is happening in the encounter of the two groups. In order to privilege an embodied understanding of knowledge, critical scholars have advocated that we view the production of scholarship through a framework of "situated knowledge" (Haraway, 1988). Therefore, I advocate that we view doulas' embodied knowledge of the child birthing process as "situated knowledge," which privileges birthing women's bodies, minds, and agencies. The "situated knowledge" on child birthing

---

[3] I explain the definition of propositional knowledge in Chapter 1 *Feminist Perspective, Body, and Epistemology.* Dalmiya and Alcoff define propositional knowledge by narrating an Indian epic *The Mahabharata.* Propositional knowledge refers to knowledge that is abstracted from a point of view and where the experience and situated location of the knowledge producer are made invisible— these women were considered ignorant.

allows for the knowledge of standpoints of women (especially pregnant women and birthing mothers) to produce knowledge and privilege connections. Along with the epistemic struggle over the knowledge of the child birthing process, the relational dialectic conflicts are also partially caused by a "different understanding of knowledge," which is similar to Qin Nan's observation. Obstetricians and midwives who graduated from medical schools with institutional scientific trainings were viewed as having "authoritative knowledge" (Davis-Floyd, 2004; Davis-Floyd & Cheyney, 2009; Jordan & Davis-Floyd, 1993; Henley, 2015). Constructed within a hierarchy of authoritative, medical knowledge, obstetrics staff and doulas occupy different positionalities, respectively, in which the former groups are treated with higher respect and authority (thus, accurate knowledge) while the latter group is viewed with lower respect and non-evidence-based knowledge. When disagreements occur between an obstetrician and/or midwife and a doula during a woman's labor, the doula must normally apologize first to resolve the conflict, in spite of whether she had made a mistake.

The unequal power dynamics determine how obstetrics staff and doulas perceive "solutions to the conflicts" in labor suites. Doulas are more likely to use moderate strategies, such as making compromises or withdrawing from arguments. Although doulas (both hospital-based doulas and mother doulas) and obstetricians and midwives are maternal health care workers, they operate within different discourses and positions in the labor suites. Instead of viewing obstetrics staff as their colleagues or coworkers, the hospital-based doulas view them as their supervisors in labor suites. Doulas intend to maintain "a harmonious" relationship with obstetrics staff most of the time.

As many news media reported, there have been many arguments, law suits, incidents of physical violence, and cyber-bullying that have occurred between patients and hospital staff, including obstetricians, nurses, midwives, and hospital managers (see Yao et al., 2014; Wang & Zhang, 2016; Hesketh et al., 2012). Relationships between patients and hospital staff are intensive. These intensive relationships reinforce the position of obstetrics staff since "everyone in the labor suites intend[s] to minimize risks" for pregnant women in labor. As one of the participants, Ai Bei—a midwife—said, "We just want to make sure both the mother and her child are safe. We just hope there is no fight." The "safe labor result" has become one of the reasons that some obstetricians and midwives practice their medical expertise but devalue or do not trust doulas' practices and assistance with pregnant women in labor.

Instead of compromising or withdrawing from relational conflicts, I suggest establishing collaborative relationships between doulas and obstetricians and/or midwives in the labor suites. Collaborative relationships would allow each group to voice their concerns and start discussions. First and foremost, both obstetrics staff and doulas should hold positive attitudes toward conflict. In my interviews, I found that sometimes doulas and obstetricians/midwives did not really communicate with each other—they assumed the other side was wrong or not good at helping pregnant women in labor. Lin Jing was welcomed in labor suites because she communicated very well with the obstetricians/midwives she worked with. In turn, the obstetricians along with midwives were more likely to be open-minded and willing to learn more about the doula care profession. Likewise, doulas' attitudes toward the expertise of obstetrics staff also are important factors in their relational dialectics.

The relational conflicts between doulas and obstetric staff represent an epistemic struggle over knowledge about the childbirth process. The conflicts were also partially caused by different conceptions of authoritative knowledge about medical interventions and the doula care profession, among other factors. Important, unequal power dynamics determined how doulas and obstetrics staff managed relational conflicts, their different attitudes toward conflict, and their problem-solving strategies. Relational conflicts are inevitable in different types of relationships. Thus, I suggest viewing doulas' embodied knowledge of the child birthing process as "situated knowledge" and constructing collaborative relationships between obstetrics staff and doulas to better help women in labor.

References

Brake, T., Walker, D. M., & Walker, T. (1995). *Doing business internationally: The guide to cross-cultural success*. McGraw Hill.

Cheung, N. F., Mander, R., & Cheng, L. (2005). The 'doula-midwives' in Shanghai. *Evidence Based Midwifery, 3*(2), 73–80.

Cheung, N. F., Mander, R., Wang, X., Fu, W., & Zhu, J. (2009). Chinese midwives' views on a proposed midwife-led normal birth unit. *Midwifery, 25*(6), 744–755. https://doi.org/10.1016/j.midw.2009.03.008

Dalmiya, V., & Alcoff, L. (1993). Are 'old wives tales' justified. In L. Alcoff & E. Potter (Eds.), *Feminist Epistemologies*. New York: Routledge.

Davis-Floyd, R. E. (2004). *Birth as an American rite of passage: With a new preface*. University of California Press. https://doi.org/10.1525/j.ctt1pndwn

Davis-Floyd, R. E., & Cheyney, M. (2009). Birth and the big bad wolf: an evolutionary perspective. In H. Selin & P. K. Stone (Eds.), *Childbirth across cultures* (pp. 1–22). Springer.

Ehrenreich, B., & English, D. (2010). *Witches, midwives, & nurses: A history of women healers*. The Feminist Press at CUNY, New York.

Guerrero, L. K., Andersen, P. A., & Afifi, W. A. (2011). *Close encounters: Communication in relationships* (3rd ed.). Sage.

Haraway, D. (1988). Situated knowledges: The science question in feminism and the privilege of partial perspective. *Feminist Studies, 14*(3), 575–599. https://doi.org/10.2307/3178066

Henley, M. M. (2015). Alternative and authoritative knowledge: The role of certification for defining expertise among doulas. *Social Currents, 2*(3), 260–279. https://doi.org/10.1177/2329496515589851

Hesketh, T., Wu, D., Mao, L., & Ma, N. (2012). Violence against doctors in China. *British Medical Journal, 345*, e5730. https://doi.org/10.1136/bmj.e5730

Jordan, B., & Davis-Floyd, R. (1993). *Birth in four cultures: A crosscultural investigation of childbirth in Yucatan*. In *Holland, Sweden, and the United States*. Waveland Press.

Towler, J., & Bramall, J. (1986). *Midwives in history and society*. Taylor & Francis.

Verderber, K. S., & MacGeorge, E. L. (2016). *Inter-act: Interpersonal communication concepts, skills, and contexts* (14th ed.). Oxford University Press.

Wang, S., & Zhang, X. (2016). Both doctors and patients are victims in China. *International Journal of Cardiology, 223*, 289–289. https://doi.org/10.1016/j.ijcard.2016.07.286

Yao, S., Zeng, Q., Peng, M., Ren, S., Chen, G., & Wang, J. (2014). Stop violence against medical workers in China. *Journal of Thoracic Disease, 6*(6), E141–E145. https://doi.org/10.3978/j.issn.2072-1439.2014.06.10

Chapter 6
Looking Forward

Chinese doulas started to work as a group of women to advocate for women's respectful maternity healthcare in labor. Some of the doulas I interviewed said they started this work to resist the medicalization of women's bodies and to empower women, as well as forming supportive groups (both on- and offline). As I elaborated in the previous chapters, doulas have become a unique group of maternal healthcare workers in the contemporary Chinese maternity system. Different from obstetricians, nurses, and midwives, who have been recognized as maternal healthcare workers nationwide, Chinese doulas are an emerging group. In terms of the future development of doula care in China, this group faces both opportunities and challenges.

Continuing Development in Chinese Doula Care Work

Many Chinese doulas in this study talked about future directions of the doula profession and the promotion of doula care in China. Shen Yu, a hospital-based doula, said that "doula as a profession and a childbirth worker advocating for natural birth was just introduced to mainland China less than a decade ago." Across the nation, not many maternity hospitals provide doula care in labor. "Fewer hospitals allow private doulas (or mother doulas) to enter in the delivery rooms," Shen Yu said. She also explained that time and effort are the challenges Chinese women face to become professional doulas. Shen Yu said,

> To become a certified doula, it requires a lot of effort and financial investment. Doulas took time to participate in different courses or seminars, and doulas had to pass different tests (both international and national).

Meanwhile, Qin Nan, an obstetrician and doula, suggested that most obstetricians and midwives working at tier-one cities' maternal hospitals had a general understanding of doulas and doula care in childbirth because these groups of obstetrics staff were "always on the cutting edge of the maternal knowledge." Therefore, the promotion of doulas and doula care would be easier in tier-one cities, where the hospital leaders/managers might be more inclined to promote the doula care system.

© The Author(s), under exclusive license to Springer Nature Switzerland AG 2021   67
Z. Z. Dai, *Maternal Healthcare and Doulas in China*,
https://doi.org/10.1007/978-3-030-46963-4_6

On the other hand, there were some challenges for the promotion of doulas and doula care in some tier-two cities' maternal hospitals. Qin Nan stated,

> Obstetrics staff who work in tier-two cities might not know doulas and doula care. In my opinion, there are many problems with the promotion of maternal health for the public in tier-two cities. To some extent, we fail in promoting the ideas of respectful maternal healthcare and healthy pregnancy.

Yue Le, an experienced midwife, explained her observation of the challenges that Chinese maternal hospitals encounter with doulas and doula care development. Yue Le explained,

> In my opinion, one of the difficulties is the shortage of obstetrics staff in the delivery rooms. One delivery room only has three or four midwives, but it will have about 20 expectant women in labor. It is impossible to ask our midwives to provide doula care for every single expectant woman in labor.

However, Yue Le added, "If the public maternity hospitals would accept private doulas or train hospital-based doulas, that would bring some bright sides to the promotion of doula care."

Similarly, Qin Nan commented on the development of the doula profession in China. She said,

> We can treat the doula profession as a new commercial product just appearing on the market. Hiring a doula for women in childbirth is quite new in China, and it definitely takes time for Chinese women and their families to accept doulas and doula care.

Future Development of Doula Care in China

Many Chinese doulas expressed their opinions about the future development of the doula profession. Some of the participants talked about the bright side or their positive attitudes toward doula promotion programs in the contemporary Chinese maternal healthcare system. For instance, Qin Nan, who was highly involved with doula professional development and organized several seminars and talks nationally, saw high potential for development of the doula profession. She believed that "doula care developed while accompanying the national economy's progress." As Qin Nan said, "There will be a large potential market for both doulas and pregnant women."

At the same time, many challenges may hinder the development of doula care in China. It took time for both current obstetricians, midwives, and pregnant women's families to accept the new idea of doula care in contemporary maternal hospitals. Through the interviews I had with Chinese doulas, I learned that many private hospitals were more likely to welcome doulas and doula care for women in labor. Many of the participants (especially mother doulas) mentioned that they were more likely to be allowed to work in labor suites in private hospitals. Chinese public hospitals were more likely to train current registered nurses, midwives, and obstetricians to be doulas. After they receive relevant doula care training provided by the hospitals, the obstetrics staff started to practice doula care for laboring mothers. A hospital-based doula also needed to prepare for routine medical practice for vaginal births.

One of the reasons that Chinese certified nurses or midwives have acted as doulas was because lots of public hospitals (government-based) did not allow non-obstetrics staff to enter the delivery rooms (Raven et al., 2015; Cheung et al., 2005). In fact, neither a woman's family members nor other birth companions were allowed to be with her in the delivery room to provide support to her during vaginal birth since the labor suite was shared by many other laboring mothers and was considered too crowded to accommodate other birth companions (Cheung et al., 2005). Different from the restrictions in the public maternity hospitals, private hospitals are more flexible and are open to allowing a birthing mother's families and her doula to enter the labor suite. As I examined in the previous chapters, private hospitals make their own management decisions and fully take responsibility for profits and losses. Likewise, allowing professional doulas in the labor suites to provide continuous support for women in labor would increase doula care, a maternity healthcare profession, prevalent among pregnant women and their families. Private maternity hospitals, therefore, provide an opportunity for doulas to practice their maternity healthcare services with birthing mothers, which also support private hospitals' profits from an economic perspective.

However, there are obvious differences regarding how women in different social classes access maternity healthcare resources (e.g., maternity hospitals, healthcare workers). In my field study, I observed that Chinese middle-class pregnant women are more likely to have financial resources to labor in a private hospital and to hire private doulas to support their labor processes. For instance, a woman has to pay at least RMB 10,000[1] if she delivers her child at WeCare WMH. Since WeCare WMH provides hospital-based doulas for birthing mothers, mothers will not have to pay an extra fee for doulas. However, birthing mothers have to pay extra money for doulas in many other private maternity hospitals. The price of natural delivery at a government-based hospital is about RMB 3000[2] (or even less). A woman and her family's socioeconomic status directly impact her choice of birthing hospitals. If the doula care support for birthing women only occurs in private hospitals, does it mean that women are allowed self-determination based on their different socioeconomic statuses?

Further, the provision of doula care comes at a higher premium for pregnant women and their families. Not everyone is able to or would like to pay an additional fee for doula care in labor. Just as He Pei said, "The doula care fee will not be covered by women's maternal health insurance. The cost would be a financial burden

---

[1] RMB 10,000 equals $1572 (USD). RMB 10,000 is only for women who labor in natural birth. If a woman ends up with C-section, the price will be much higher. WeCare WMH also charges different prices based on the wards that a woman chooses. The price of natural delivery ranges from RMB 10,000 to RMB 37,000. Another private hospital, United Family Hospital and Clinics, charges about RMB 56,000 ($8,800) for women who have natural delivery.

[2] RMB 3000 equals $470 (USD).

for many families." Therefore, the development of doula care might involve reforms to Chinese insurance policies or related adjustments in terms of reimbursement.

In fact, Chinese maternal hospitals encourage doulas and doula care development. Private maternity hospitals are more likely to encourage mother doulas to work with pregnant women in the delivery rooms, while public hospitals are more likely to train their own registered childbirth educators, nurses, midwives, and obstetricians to be hospital-based doulas. As a new profession in contemporary Chinese society, doula care has taken time to gain recognition and acceptance among Chinese women, their families, and obstetricians and midwives.

References

Cheung, N. F., Mander, R., & Cheng, L. (2005). The 'doula-midwives' in Shanghai. *Evidence Based Midwifery, 3*(2), 73–80.

Raven, J., van den Broek, N., Tao, F., Kun, H., & Tolhurst, R. (2015). The quality of childbirth care in China: women's voices: A qualitative study. *BMC Pregnancy and Childbirth, 15*(1), 113. Retrieved from https://bmcpregnancychildbirth.biomedcentral.com/articles/10.1186/s12884-015-0545-9

Chapter 7
Concluding Thoughts and a New Beginning

The project in this book was broadly focused around the examination of the emergence of a "doula" phenomenon and the role that doula care workers play in for Chinese women during pregnancy and childbirth. I have produced particular situated interpretations and suggestions, in this project, based on evidence gathered through interviews and scholarly observations. All of these are guided by women-centered approach and health communication perspectives. This project is a start. Further conversations and research on women, women's bodies, and maternity healthcare in health communication are called for.

In this project, I explored the career motivations and working experiences of Chinese doula workers and their interactions with pregnant women, obstetricians, and midwives. Chinese doula workers empower birthing mothers by providing "situated knowledge" in the process that some women are making or owning choices. However, these women are more likely to be economically privileged. Many Chinese doulas are also aware of these contradictions, and they continue working for pregnant women or birthing mothers because they still carry hope and faith in doula care.

I also examined the sisterhood and close friendships that Chinese doulas established with pregnant women through the provision of different kinds of support; Chinese doulas' perceptions of natural birth and medical interventions; relational conflicts they encountered in their work and with healthcare staff; and their thoughts about the ongoing development of the doula care profession in China. Chinese doulas, as a group of emerging maternity healthcare workers, advocate for the resistance of medical authoritative knowledge by placing women's bodies, emotions, and ideas at the center of decision making. I also raised questions in relation to the maternity healthcare that doulas provide for women in labor and shared concerns about the management of doulas' emotions by referencing emotional labour theory.

There are other possible approaches for conducting this type of research, and there are potential ways to improve this study. In this final chapter, I reflect on the work that has been done and look forward to what can be done in the future. I also interweave my research findings with family stories and scholarly reflections on the whole project.

Z. Z. Dai, *Maternal Healthcare and Doulas in China*,
https://doi.org/10.1007/978-3-030-46963-4_7

Family Stories: *30 Years Ago, and After*

I was born in the late 1980s. In discussion with my mother, I learned that when my mother was pregnant about 30 years ago she and my father did not have any access to childbirth education classes in the community clinics. In those days, there was no childbirth education, nor were there community organizations that could be consulted for advice and information. Although my mother graduated from a medical school and had worked as a general physician at a hospital, she was not quite sure what to expect in childbirth.

Through the years, my mother repeatedly told me that the scientific medical knowledge she learned from medical school was not very helpful to her when she herself went into labor. She was well educated in both physiology and pathology, but her body had been seemingly "out of her control" as she was giving birth to a child. "The knowledge I learned was not very helpful, and I could not use any physiological knowledge to guide my own labor," she said. One of the few guides my mother had for this embodied experience was my grandmother—her mother in-law. My grandmother told her,

> Labor is painful. You have to bear it by yourself. After hours of pain, you will deliver the baby. Every woman experiences the same thing. My mother delivered me at home, but you will labor in the hospital with help from doctors (obstetricians and midwives). Don't worry.

Initially, my mom's expected due date was November 4, but I was born one week earlier. On October 30, her water broke after dinner, and my dad sent her to the hospital immediately. Both knew that the baby was coming. Thirty years ago, fathers were not allowed to be present for their baby's birth. In fact, no one could be with the mothers, neither her husband nor her parents.

My mom was there lying on the bed of the delivery room by herself. Her husband was not there nor were her other immediate family members. My mother recalled that almost four or five other pregnant women were in the delivery room that night, and only a couple of midwives and one obstetrician were on duty. All the midwives and obstetrician were so busy that they were not able to give adequate attention to each expectant mother.

While my mom was in labor, the midwives and the obstetrician asked her to "push hard," but she said she did not know how to do it. According to my mother's narratives, it took about 10 hours for her to be done with childbirth. It was worth noting that my mom referred to one of the midwives as an "older sister midwife." My mom said,

> She was a senior midwife, and she reminded me of my older sister. The "older sister midwife" was actually the one who helped me to deliver you. I was a bit worried about you…, but she was very experienced. She was the one told me, "OK, it is full dilation. Ready to go! Push hard!"

As a mother, she wanted to see and touch her baby. The "sister midwife" informed her of the sex—a baby girl.[1] "Look, it is a girl. I am going to inform your husband," the midwife said. It is forbidden for expectant Chinese parents to do a sex test before a child's birth. This law is designed to prevent Chinese parents from aborting their babies if they knew the baby would be female (Ma, 2013; Zhang, 2008; Loh & Remick, 2015). Hence, the first thing a mother learns about her newborn baby is the sex: boy or girl.

Further, the midwife took the baby girl (me) to a room with other newborns. After several hours, my mom had me by her side—eventually. We had skin-to-skin touch for the first time in our lives. Although I was personally involved in my mother's labor, I only learned about her labor stories as she shared them with me in the past several years. One of my initial, personal motivations to complete this project on women's childbirth experiences was because of my mother and her experience. As she mentioned, labor was a long process during which she experienced feelings of hopelessness, isolation, but also fulfilled with lots of happiness. She said,

> When I first heard you cry, I knew you were delivered safely. You were healthy so that made all the suffering and pain worthwhile. I was happy when I knew you were delivered and that you were healthy.

It is important to point out that my mother was neither the first nor the only mother who had expressed the sentiment, "Once the child was healthy, I was fine." Many of my female family members, friends, and colleagues in different generations and sociocultural backgrounds expressed the same idea: women in labor can sacrifice everything just to achieve one goal—the baby's safety.

Fortunately, information about childbirth is much more accessible to my generation. Childbirth has become a topic discussed among families, friends, and the media. Expectant parents of my generation in China can access information about childbirth from the hospitals where the mothers plan to deliver their babies. For instance, AMCARE Women and Children's Health Hospital and United Family Healthcare[2] offer weekly and/or monthly childbirth education classes, which are open and free to the public. Sometimes, a few maternity hospitals organize informative seminars and activities for expectant parents. These public talks and activities normally cover several topics, including what pregnant women can eat during the pregnancy, what kind of exercise pregnant women can do, what husbands can do for their pregnant wives, introduction to breastfeeding, and more. Meanwhile, a large number of firsthand birth stories can now be read on various social media platforms

---

[1] Regarding Chinese physicians/midwives in this study, they often use the terms "gender" and "sex" with the same meanings. I use the term "sex" here to describe a boy or girl's biological profile.

[2] AMCARE Women and Children's Hospital is an international private maternity hospital. It was established in 2004 by AMCARE hospital group. There are eight affiliated hospitals/clinics in mainland China. More information can be retrieved from: http://www.amcare.com.cn. United Family Healthcare is an international-level health system. Since 1997, it has established 14 satellite clinics and medical centers in China. More information can be retrieved from http://ufh.com.cn/

in China. Likewise, there is a growing number of Chinese media platforms providing information for people to understand pregnancy and childbirth, including television programs, books, newspapers, and the Internet (e.g., Mama Website, Yama Website, the Chinese social media Weibo account of "Question & Answers with Obstetricians," the social media WeChat account of "Mitu Childbirth"[3]).

I approached this project focused on doulas among Chinese maternity healthcare workers and adopted women-centered approach and health communication frameworks by engaging discussions around women's bodies during pregnancy and childbirth. As a health communication researcher and a person who grew up in China, my standpoint (Harding, 1993) allows me to study the phenomena of doula care in China as a communication researcher embedded in the culture and language rather than as an outsider. Straddling both the Western academy and the Chinese culture also allows me a certain kind of epistemic in-between and a "double-vision" (Narayan, 2004) that also sheds light on how a larger global movement toward midwifery shapes the particular case of Chinese doulas. Thus, I have looked at emerging contexts of midwifery—referred to as 'doula care"—and how these doula workers are an emerging group of maternity healthcare workers. Doula care phenomenon, as it emerges as a viable profession for women in China, reveals nuances and contradictions and lends itself to an examination through a critical health communication lens and a relational communication perspective.

As I write this project, I cannot help thinking about my mother's pregnancy and childbirth experiences, and the other women in her generation, in comparison with women in my generation. I ask myself,

How would *she* feel if *she* were to experience labor today?
If *she* were to experience labor today, would *she* feel different if *her husband or family members* could enter the labor suite with *her*?
If *she* were to experience labor today, would *she* have a doula?
In a labor suite, what changes have been made in the past three decades?

Frankly, as many of my female family members and friends gave birth to their children recent years, I have witnessed a significant change in the labor suite (regarding obstetric staff arrangement, respectful maternity healthcare, labor suite equipment, and delivery room interior design) comparing to the one that I was born into three decades ago. Last year (2019), one of my interviewees shared with me a few pictures of LDR room from her current workplace. She told me,

LDR refers labor, delivery, recovery and postpartum room. It is an advanced equipped room that a woman can remain in the same room throughout the birthing experience and into the postpartum period.

I am happy for my interviewee(s) who can work in this kind of advanced equipped labor suite, and I am happier for the women who are able to choose to have these LDR rooms and with a doula-supported laboring experience.

---

[3] Mama Website retrieved from: www.mama.cn; Yama Website retrieved from: www.yanma.com; Weibo account of Question &Answer with Obstetricians retrieved from: https://weibo.com/5860115721/; WeChat account of "Mitu Childbirth" retrieved from #metoo201608.

As I have noted throughout this project, it has been a humbling experience for me to recognize that this interdisciplinary project is not merely to satisfy the requirement of a doctoral degree. Doulas and doula care have become high-profile symbols in the discourses about maternal healthcare in contemporary China. The discourse about doulas and the doula care profession in China is inseparable from the discourse of women's bodies, reproduction, motherhood, and breastfeeding, as well as overall health. The connection between these discourses motivates me to contribute my scholarship toward the future of Chinese women's maternity healthcare.

A New Beginning

To end the writing of this project, I would like to reflect some of my thoughts. Research for this book was originated from a research project that I have started to work on since early 2017. By the time this book is about to finish, it has been 2020 already. Through the years, both of my professional and personal life have been dramatically changed. Right now, we are in the middle of a global pandemic. Pregnant women and their families might face unimaginable challenges and questions during pregnancy as well as the birth process. As a health communication researcher, my current project is focusing on understanding pregnancy and birth during the coronavirus crisis. By saying that, it is important to point out that my scholarly research and personal understanding for doulas and maternity healthcare have been developed and explored since 2017.

As a health communication researcher with the interpretive paradigm, my writing for the research project was influenced (still is influenced and will be influenced) by my professional and individual experience. In other words, the perception and understanding for a research project is not fixed but in a fluid status. Moreover, it is significant to point out that the maternity healthcare in China, along with doula care profession and doula support for women, has progressively developed. It will be unfair to discuss doula care program and doula profession in China without a holistic and integrated consideration from a national aspect. Also, every single doula as well as all obstetric staff should be awarded for credits to honor their love, passion, dedication, and professionalism to their career and maternity healthcare in general.

One of my close academic sisters asked me, "If you have a second chance to rewrite this project, will you do it?" Frankly, my answer is *yes*. Looking back to my writings from 2017 to 2018, I certainly recognized the limitations and incomplete aspects of the research. First, the sample size of participants is not very big, and broad generalizations cannot be made. Most of the participants in this study work in urban areas in China, which differ from rural China, for example, in terms of socioeconomics. Thus, a future research extension of this work could include a comparative study between Chinese doulas in urban and rural areas.

Moreover, this study focuses on Chinese doulas' professional development in terms of doulas' career motivations, their construction of sisterhood and close friendships with expectant mothers, their different attitudes about medical and technological interventions, their negotiation of conflict with obstetricians and midwives regarding authoritative knowledge, and their thoughts on the future development of the doula care profession in China. Like Ai Bei, an experienced midwife, said,

> Chinese and American women have different physical body types. For instance, we eat a lot of vegetables and they (Americans) probably eat meat and dairy. We are different. The practice of maternity healthcare will be different too.

Therefore, future studies could perform a comparative analysis of the motivations of doula workers in the United States and China, as well as studies examining the medical and cultural contexts in both countries. Comparison studies that adopt an intercultural communication perspective would enrich the scholarship on maternal healthcare and reproductive healthcare in general.

As I found in this project, many participants utilize social media (e.g., WeChat, Weibo) as the digital platform to construct supportive community groups involving doulas, pregnant women, and families. Future studies could explore the construction of digital supportive communities between doulas and pregnant women. In particular, for mother doulas who own their businesses, it will be important to study how they pursue entrepreneurship and establish and develop their businesses via social media or related media platforms. It is interesting to mention that after conducting interviews with many professional doulas we exchanged numbers as well as social media accounts. Through the years, I have observed their activities on different social media platforms, in which I have witnessed their professional growth and training development. Some of them started to have their own business, some of them participated in a few more doula-related training workshops, and some of them wrote and published their own doula profession experiences. Once again, I appreciate all of them gave me a chance to interview them and document their stories.

Further, there are many American doulas and/or childbirth educators (e.g., Penny Smikin, Jeanette Crenshaw, Michele Ondeck, Linda Smith, Barbara Harper, Tamela Hatcher) who have visited China to provide seminars and participate in different childbirth education activities. Also, my friend Shujuan and the "Mitu team" have organized various childbirth education activities across the nation, including one Lamaze Childbirth Education seminar in Shenzhen and a Sound Birthing Music workshop in Xuzhou, among others. It would be beneficial to hear American doula workers' voices about the doula care profession's development in China. Future studies could adopt an intercultural health communication approach to focus on American doula workers, who have had rich experiences and interactions with Chinese doulas as well as personally observed and participated in the development of Chinese doula care.

"Childbirth knowledge is comprised of both biological knowledge of pregnancy and labor and social knowledge" (Lazarus, 1994, p. 26). Women in different socioeconomic backgrounds have various understandings about childbirth knowledge, which also have impacts on women's abilities to act on such knowledge (Lazarus,

1988, 1994). Meanwhile, there are obvious differences in the access women from different social classes have to maternity healthcare resources. At WeCare WMH, I have observed that Chinese middle-class pregnant women are more likely to have financial abilities to hire private doulas to support their labor processes and employ a lactation consultant to receive related service on breastfeeding. A middle-class Chinese woman is even able to stay in a postpartum care center (*yuezi huisuo* in Chinese) for about 30 days to receive some postpartum caring from professional maternal healthcare workers. The cost range of postpartum healthcare is around RMB 20,000 to RMB 80,000.[4] Therefore, it is important to give voice to Chinese women about their pregnancy and childbearing experiences; I would like to hear their voice on doula care, as well as their experiences of interactions with maternal healthcare workers. Through the entire project, I saw that Chinese doulas create some promising respectful maternity healthcare practices in the labor suite. At the minimum, doulas can continue to play a key role as maternal healthcare activists by advocating for and prioritizing women's bodies and feelings. There is no doubt that Chinese doulas are an emerging group of female health caregivers who advocate for and bring about women's empowerment in pregnancy and childbirth.

References

Harding, S. (1993). Rethinking standpoint epistemology: "What is strong objectivity"? In L. Alcoff & E. Potter (Eds.), *Feminist epistemology* (pp. 49–92). Routledge.

Lazarus, E. S. (1988). Poor women, poor outcomes: Social class and reproductive health. *Childbirth in America: Anthropological Perspectives*, 39–54.

Lazarus, E. S. (1994). What do women want?: Issues of choice, control, and class in pregnancy and childbirth. *Medical Anthropology Quarterly, 8*(1), 25–46.

Loh, C., & Remick, E. (2015). China's skewed sex ratio and the one-child policy. *China Quarterly, 222*, 295–319. https://doi.org/10.1017/S0305741015000375

Ma, J. (2013, May 21). China's brutal one-child policy. *The New York Times*. Retrieved from https://www.nytimes.com/2013/05/22/opinion/chinas-brutal-one-child-policy.html

Narayan, U. (2004). The project of feminist epistemology: Perspectives from a nonwestern feminist. In S. G. Harding (Ed.), *The feminist standpoint theory reader: Intellectual and political controversies* (pp. 213–224). Routledge.

Wong, O. M. H. (2016). The changing relationship of women with their natal families. *Journal of Sociology, 52*(1), 53–67. https://doi.org/10.1177/1440783315587797

Zhang, Y. (2008). *Layered motherhood for Chinese mother bloggers: A feminist Foucauldian analysis*. Doctoral dissertation, Bowling Green State University, Bowling Green, OH. Retrieved from ProQuest.

---

[4] RMB 20,000 equals $3143; RMB 80,000 equals $12,573 (both USD).

Index

Printed in the United States
by Baker & Taylor Publisher Services